FOPLA / AABPO

1

# The
# DISH DIET<sup>SM</sup>

## WATCH YOUR PLATE
## NOT YOUR WEIGHT

*Roberta Cahn, BSChE & MSBio-ChE*
*Danuta Highet, BSME & MM*

*Illustrations by Stephanie Snyder*

*Maidin Works*
*Voorhees, NJ*

*This book is dedicated to every person*

*who ever had to diet to lose weight.*

# Table of Contents

# Table of Contents

# Preface

You have picked up this book because you or someone you know is coping with fighting the battle of the bulge. You are not alone. Obesity is growing in the United States and many other countries around the world at an astonishing rate. The authors have been fighting the battle themselves and watching their friends and family members lose to the overpowering force of this wave. Their concern is for our society today as well as the future generations that will follow us.

The authors looked to the past to see how we got to where we are today as individuals and as a society. They also envisioned the future if we continue on the current path. They did not like what they saw and have made it their mission to help reverse this trend.

They focused their energy on the things we can do today to change the direction we are heading. They looked for small changes that we all can make to put ourselves and our society on the path to being fit and fulfilled. They came to the conclusion that we need to revolutionize how we eat. As a result, they developed a patent pending method for sizing and using dishware to help people lose weight, keep it off, and even prevent becoming overweight to start with. Now you can easily change how much you eat without changing what you eat, and succeed in losing weight and keeping it off permanently.

# Introduction

*"Today is the first day of the rest of your life."* [1]
Charles Dederich

Life is a journey. At any point in time, you can look back to see how you got here. You can examine where you are and predict where you will be in the future. Check the present to see if you are happy where you are. Try to envision the future if you stay on the current path. Can you see the possibilities that await you if you could make small changes in how you live today?

The past is done. No matter how much you think about it and wish you could change it, you can't. But you can learn from it, and most importantly, you can learn what you did *right*.

Looking at the past actions you took may be the key to getting you on the path to success. It can help you decide what you need to do more of, to do less of, to start or stop doing altogether. So look to the past to help you answer the question, "What do I do going forward?"

You will probably find that there are many aspects of your life which you are happy about. Do not change those!

Now ask yourself, "Are there things that I can do to improve my quality of life, to make it better, easier, and more fulfilling?"

That's the beauty of living. There are always things we can do better. For the aspects of your life you like, you can stay on the current path. For the aspects of your life you *don't* like, you can plan today to put yourself on the path to where you want to be. You can change your future by changing what you do at the present. Every step you take today is putting you on the path to your future. If you do not like where you're going, you have the power to change these steps to shift to where you want to be.

You have a choice! You can look back at your past and feel disappointment and regret. On the other hand, you can look back to find a treasury of knowledge. Your past contains the information that can help you make changes today to get you on a new path towards a healthy and happy future.

It doesn't take giant leaps to get you on the right path. Every small step in the right direction gets you closer to where you want to be. There are things you can do to make this journey easier. There will be times when you will stray from your path. The only way to succeed is to get right back on it.

No matter who you are, you are capable of making changes. These may be small changes at first, but they can result in great rewards. Start focusing on what you can do, and in the end you may surprise even yourself with what you are capable of achieving.

Next look at your recent past. Think about your lifestyle last month or last week. Chances are that you will not remember when and what you ate. Starting a diary may prove to be helpful in figuring out your daily/weekly "eating journey."

Examine your trip from Monday to Sunday. What made you feel that you needed to eat? What triggered you to think about food? Were you really hungry, or was there food in front of you? Was it time to eat, or did a commercial tempt you? Did you pass by a fast food restaurant or a vending machine? Did you see someone else eating? Something triggered you to want food and get food.

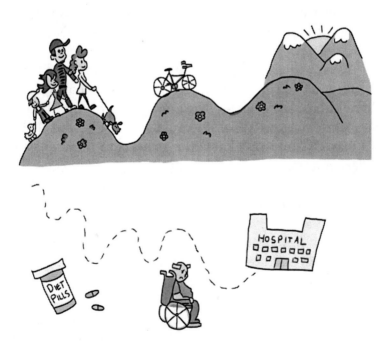

*It's a matter of life and health. Choose your path forward.*

17

You also make your own decisions regarding when to stop eating at any given point in time. What made you stop? Was it the pain in your stomach? Did you need to open the button on your slacks or loosen up your belt? Did you run out of food, or reach the bottom of a package? Did you have to go back to work? Or maybe you just didn't want to get up for more. Knowing when you stop eating is another important factor that will help you stay healthy. You will be able to figure out how to stop sooner so you eat less.

This information will help you to make changes to get on the path you want for your future. It will aid you in identifying your strengths and your weaknesses. This book will show you how to use that knowledge to reach your goals.

What will also help you stay on your path is to envision the future. First, envision what your future will be like if you do not make any changes. Next, imagine a future where you *do* make changes. "What if I could...? What if I did...? What if I was...?" You won't know the answers to these questions unless you try.

Your vision and your actions will determine your future. Take all the energy of yearning for what could have been and all the feelings of regret for what was lost, shake them up together, and create a potion for new life from this day forward.

Transform that negative energy into the power to motivate you to change. Start channeling this energy into making positive changes in your life. Every day is a new beginning filled with new possibilities.

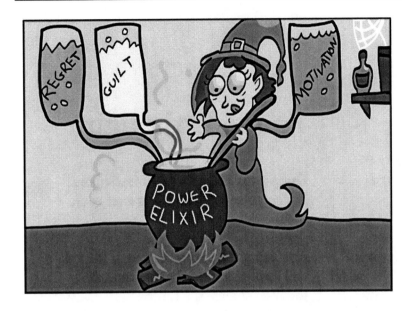

    The pace of life is speeding up. You need to arm yourself with tools that will help you to eat right and keep up. This book will provide the information you need to help you on your journey to a healthier and more rewarding life.

# Food for thought:

*Past:* Our past is a treasury of knowledge. Acceptance will help focus energy on the future success.

*Present:* Analyzing the past and current lifestyle will lead to actions that we can take today to change the future.

*Future:* Envisioning the opportunities and possibilities will help motivate us to make the changes today that lead to future rewards.

*Tools:* We need the right tools for the right job. Simple changes like changing the dishware you eat from and utensils you eat with can help you succeed.

*Change:* Small gradual steps are easier and more effective in the long-term.

# Part 1:

# The Past - Knowledge

# Chapter 1

# How Did We Get Here?

*"Learn from the past in order to improve the present, and to better shape the future."* [2]

Ferdowsi

Our families, our neighbors, and our friends are getting bigger and bigger, and so are we. We believe we are eating the same way as we always have, so WHY ARE WE GAINING WEIGHT?

We don't mean big like in the old days. What used to be considered "big" is now considered average. When we were kids we almost never saw anyone who was "morbidly obese." Yet now, not a day goes by when we don't see someone struggle to get onto a bus or into a car, climb a set of stairs, or even just sit comfortably in a chair.

One of the reasons we are not able to get at the obesity problem is that we confuse being obese with being *morbidly* obese. We also have a difficult time talking about it because there is a social stigma associated with this term.

Therefore, we camouflage it by referring to ourselves as "big." This and many other factors are contributing to the increase of obesity rates.

The trends are scary. In many states in the United States, one out of three people is obese. That means if you live in one of these locations and you have two friends sitting with you, chances are that one of you is obese. If you do not live in one of these locations you might think "I am safe!" But you're not. Obesity can be socially contagious. It is sweeping over our nation like a wave, taking our children and their future with it. In the past 30 years the diet industry has exploded without any positive impact on stopping or reversing this disturbing surge.

What is causing this disturbing trend? Is it pollution in the air? Is it some new chemical in our drinking water?

**Possible Causes:**

- The person?
- The environment?
- The society?
- The TV commercials?
- The manufacturers?
- The media?
- The government?

**All of the above!**

There are many reasons why we are becoming more and more overweight. First, we have lost our sense of how much food we really need to live. The abundance of high fat and high calorie foods surrounding us makes us think that we can have it all. Well, we can't, and there is a huge price to pay when we try to.

The price is the loss of our health, energy, and ability to have fun. We pay the price in suffering from heart disease, diabetes, strokes, cancer, etc. We pay the price when we experience lower self image and confidence, and an increase in depression. As a result, we no longer have energy to do the things we crave and enjoy.

So how did we get here? Well, we got here because we believed that as long as we continued doing what we did in the past, we would stay as healthy as we used to be. We trusted our parents, our government, the media and our own brain!

## WE WERE DECEIVED!

Of course, it wasn't intentional. Our parents mislead us when they told us that we must finish everything on our plate. They had no idea that the plate can affect how much we eat. They did not realize that someday there would be fast food. They could not predict the "supersizing" of everything that we touched. They taught us to be frugal and always get our money's worth. "Buy bigger packages, they give you better deals," they said. They had no idea that in the long run, the cash we could have spent lounging on a tropical isle would instead be spent in the snack and soda aisle.

The government misleads us when it tells us to have a serving of this and a serving of that. They don't give us a warning in big letters that:

# A package is not a serving!

They do not tell us that we can't have a serving of chocolate, a serving of popcorn and a serving of... at the same time. There is no warning on the label of cookies that says "If you have one serving, you are going to crave more and more, and you will not stop until the package is emptied to the last crumb!"

The media tricks us every day when they constantly blast us with food commercials especially late at night. They use gimmicks to make the food seem more appealing. We listen to the promises of the commercials for exercise equipment that will let us effortlessly get back in shape. We buy these gadgets, but now we need to find hours of time just to burn the equivalent of one candy bar a day.

The stores mislead us when they stock their snack racks overflowing with packages that are ready to jump into our carts. They deceive us when they place healthy foods in some obscure section of the store. Have you ever stood in line at the register and been right next to fresh carrots or apples? What are the chances that you were staring instead at chocolate bars or candy?

Restaurants deceive us when they serve us a meal. Some pump in aromas of freshly baked cookies to make us hungrier. The more food we order, the more money they make. The more food they serve in one portion, the more likely we will return because we feel as though we got a bargain. They want us to think that a four course meal is what everyone needs to survive. They fill our plates with lots of carbs so we feel satisfied. They will offer us one-size-fits-all portions and charge us the same amount whether we weigh 110 pounds or 300 pounds.

Last but not least, **OUR BRAIN LIES!** Yes, our own brain that we have trusted for years lies to us! Our brain communicates with our hands. Our hands deliver the food to our mouth. Our brain estimates how much food we gave it yesterday and says that's how much we need today.

The day after Thanksgiving dinner it says, "Hey, I need at least as much as you gave me yesterday!" Our brain tells our eyes to look at the dish we are using. Our eyes say "I see space; there is room for more!" Our brain quickly sends the message to our hands: "Fill it up, remember when you did not get enough food two years ago. Remember how I cramped your stomach and made you feel like you were going to pass out? I can do this again!" This message bypasses our logic, since it goes right after our emotions and we immediately oblige and fill up the plate.

We lie to ourselves. "I will only have a few of these nuts." "I will exercise later today, later this week." "I can go to a buffet and just eat a small plate of veggies." "I deserve this, I had a tough day."

**"I want to enjoy my life!" is the biggest lie of them all!**

Excess weight will not bring any joy and is guaranteed to bring tons of misery. Here are some of the simple facts that explain how we got here:

- We eat more food than our body needs, and we store it as FAT.

- As we get heavier it's harder to exercise, so we burn fewer calories and we get FATTER.

- We eat lots of sweets, which may actually make you hungrier, and we get FATTER.

- We eat like when we were younger, though we need less now, and we get FATTER.

- We are filling up a plate, as usual, but the plates are much bigger, and we get FATTER.

- We add alcohol to our meals... The glassware is now bigger to match the dishware... We consume more alcohol and we get FATTER.

- Our utensils have gotten bigger, we eat more food per bite, consume faster, eat more, and we get FATTER.

- We are reminded of food more frequently, we eat more often, we consume more, and we get FATTER.

- We eat out a lot more, restaurants are serving family-size platters as meals...

### Should we go on?

Everything has changed. You need to stop listening to the lies and arm yourself with facts, logic and tools that will help you combat them.

**You need to change how you live to maintain your health, your energy and a joyful lifestyle.**

Now that you know how we got here, you have made the first step on your new journey. This book will help guide you through the process of changing how you eat and how you live, so you can keep up with the ever-changing environment. Sound like a lot of work and energy? It's not. It's simple, easy and life-changing!

# Food for thought:

*Past:*        We got here because of "lies" that encourage us to eat more and more.

*Present:*     Portions are bigger. Dishware, utensils and glassware are bigger and so are we.

*Future:*      The world is constantly changing. We need to constantly change and quickly adjust how we eat and how we live to keep up and stay healthy.

# Chapter 2

# How Did I Get Here?

*"People do not believe lies because they have to, but because they want to."* [3]

Malcolm Muggeridge

We all have ignored the truth and believed the lies fed to us by the media advertisements, the confusing government guidelines, the sleek packages of chips and candy, and even our brains. Only you can truly answer the question "How did I get here?" You alone have the information you need to figure this out. Only you know when you started to lose the battle of the bulge. It's time to look within and find the answers for yourself. You are not alone in this quest. We are here to help.

Think of your life thus far as a trip. If someone asked you to tell them how you got from Los Angeles to New York City, you would use a map to show them the routes you took. You would mark where you got a flat tire and had to take a detour.

You would highlight the fastest roads you traveled. Based on the information you wrote down, the next trip you plan from LA to NYC will be easier, faster and better.

So now you want to jot down how you got here. What did you do differently when you were young? How did you stay thin back then? If you were always overweight, were there times when you stopped gaining or did not gain as fast? What did you do differently from what you do now?

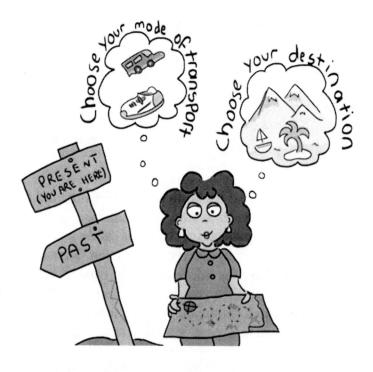

To change your life you need to examine your lifestyle, your habits, your quirks. Are you a midday binger or a night snacker?

# Chapter 2: How Did I Get Here?

Do you drive the road from work to home because it's the shortest distance, or are you mapping your route around your favorite fast food chains? Do you watch TV when you eat, or talk to friends?

Open your photo album. Check your photos and think back. You may be able to discover how your life changed you and how you changed your life to arrive where you are today. Think back and you will probably come up with some answers :

I gained 5 pounds or more after _____
(Cruise, vacation, holidays, twisted ankle, coffee house opened on my way to work, started food shopping in a warehouse style store, moved, had a baby (only women can use this excuse), got married, got divorced, placed family room next to my kitchen, put TV in my kitchen, put refrigerator and TV in my bedroom, etc.)

I lost 5 pounds or more after _____
(Joined the gym, walked Fido daily, ice cream shop closed, watched what I ate, stopped drinking alcohol, used stairs instead of elevator, played basketball, spring walks, etc.)

I snack the most when I _____

I crave food after _____

I eat well when I _____

I exercise the most when I _____

I eat the most when I _____

My greatest successes are _____

My past vices are _____

You need to think about when you were most successful. The quickest way to succeed is to do more of what helps you stay on the path. Doing more of things that you already know how to do, will make it easier and quicker to make small changes.

You need to know the bumps in the road so that you can go around them. Do you pass by a vending machine when you leave the office? Does your conversation with your friends always involve exchanging mouth-watering recipes? Are there some restaurants where you plan your dessert before you order your meals? Is "any buffet" your favorite restaurant? Is alcohol a nutrient you can't do without? Is your day ruined because you missed a white mocha?

Once you know how you got here and know your virtues and your vices you can evaluate the next step. You can plan out the small steps that are going to be the easiest to take. Changing the size of your dishware will be one of the easiest and quickest steps to implement. (See Chapter 6 "Can a Plate Affect My Weight?") When you make these changes in small increments they will painlessly get you on the right path. You will instantly feel successful and you will teach your brain who is the boss.

You will be empowered to tell your brain that the feelings it's reacting to will pass. You will have facts and logic to help you master the ability to see through the lies and through the marketing tricks and gimmicks. You will know that investing in yourself and your health is the best investment you can make. You'll be able to gradually transform yourself to be the best that you can be.

**Success breeds success.**
**Small steps can lead to big results!**

# Food for thought:

**Search:**    Describe your lifestyle when you were thinner. What did you do then that you don't do now? What didn't you do then that you do now?

**Your Success:** When did you maintain your weight? When did you lose weight? When did you feel in the best condition of your life?

**Your Vices:**  What caused you to gain excess weight?

**You Can:**    If you succeed even for a day, you have succeeded! You know it's possible!

# Chapter 3

# Fatty Buddy Is Not Your Friend

*"We are what we repeatedly do.
Excellence, then, is not an act, but a habit."* [4]
Aristotle

We all need food to survive. Every three to four hours throughout the day we need to refuel. Our bodies are similar to a car. Periodically you take the car to a gas station to refuel. Every car gives you different efficiency depending on the type of driving you do. For example, miles per gallon in the city will be lower than on a highway.

Our bodies, just like cars, are all different. We will burn food calories differently throughout the day and week depending on what activities we are involved in. As a car gets older, the engine parts wear out and the car becomes less and less efficient.

You fill up your car and periodically check how much fuel you have left. Usually, you don't think about it until you are close to being on empty. When you fill up your car, you fill up the tank. You would not buy excess gas to store in your trunk or back seat. But if you did to your car the same thing that you do to your body, every time you stopped for gas you would fill an additional container and put it in your trunk. Once your trunk was full you would put it in your back seat. After that, you would tie it to your roof, hood, etc.

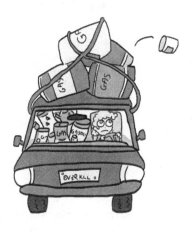

At some point the car would break down from all the weight. You would get more flat tires. Your engine and your transmission would give out.

A similar future awaits your body if you carry extra weight. If you eat the "right" amount of food, the amount that your body actually needs, you will burn it all up and have to start fresh again with your next refuel, your next meal. There is a "right" amount of food you need to live and be healthy. To keep your heart (your engine) in good shape you need to fuel with food and then burn with activity.

Every time you overeat (we don't mean eat until you have to unbuckle your pants, that's gorging not eating, we mean just eating a little more than your body needs), you store the extra that your body did not burn as fat. Historically, this ability to store fat was a good thing. When times were hard and food was scarce, you could use the extra fat to survive. But in today's world, food is not scarce, and the fat just keeps on growing and growing. So if you are following a routine of **fuel (eat) more than you burn you will store the extra**. Even if it's a small amount, your weight will keep increasing.

So every time you have a little extra snack your body does not need, you gain a little bit of weight. It takes more effort to get a container of gasoline from the back seat and pour the fuel back into your fuel tank. Similarly, it is harder for your body to get the fat back and use it as fuel. The fat keeps accumulating.

If you continue the cycle fuel-burn-store your fat will keep growing. It will grow to the point where some of us carry around the equivalent of another whole body, or more! We call this extra body fat your "Fatty-Buddy". Did you ever go to the gym and try to lift 50 or 100 pounds? Most of us cannot do that for more than a few minutes. Yet some of us carry around that much extra weight, our Fatty-Buddy, all day, every day!

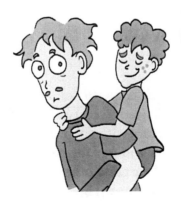

At first Fatty-Buddy is not that big. Gradually it keeps growing and growing. Everything you do starts to become more of an effort when you carry that Fatty-Buddy with you. Even standing or walking can be a chore, so imagine the workout your organs, like your heart and lungs, get every day!

Your body, just like an overloaded car, will start breaking down. Depending on how overweight you get, your organs may start failing due to the overload.

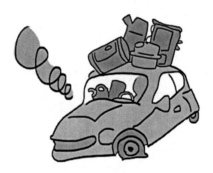

FATTY-BUDDY is not your friend! Fatty-Buddy will hurt you and keep hurting you.

Let's say someone came to you and said: "Here is your new buddy! You will need to carry and feed your buddy, take him for a walk, take him with you when you shop, go to work and go to sleep. You will pay for all the expenses that your buddy incurs. Your heart and other organs will have to work harder (for two), so your own body will "wear out" faster ..."

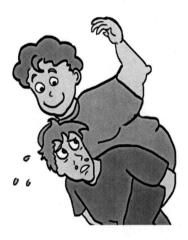

You would never agree to this! Yet gradually, snack by snack, your pal has snuck up on you and has been riding on your back ever since.

Next time you're reaching for that extra helping of food or a snack that you don't really need, stop and ask yourself, "Is this for me or for my Fatty-Buddy?"

The best way to evict the Fatty-Buddy from your body is to stop feeding him or her. If you are overweight, chances are you did not get there overnight. You gradually invited Fatty-Buddy in and kept feeding your pal. Now you have two choices. First, you can keep feeding your Fatty-Buddy and burn off all the excess calories through exercise. The more you feed your pal the more time you will need to exercise. Your second choice is to stop feeding your uninvited guest and evict him/her out of your skin. There is only room for one here!

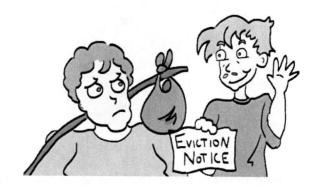

**EAT LESS - MOVE MORE
FATTY-BUDDY HAS TO GO!**

# Food for thought:

**First:**     Carrying extra fat can wear out your body parts faster.

**Second:**     Fatty-Buddy is not your friend.

**Third:**     You can lose weight if you burn more than you eat.

**Fourth:**     You can lose weight if you eat less than you burn.

**Fifth:**     Just as your Fatty-Buddy took over your body slowly and gradually, you can slowly and gradually shrink and evict your Fatty-Buddy for good.

# Chapter 4

# Your Brain Lies

*"The greatest obstacle to discovery is not ignorance - it is the illusion of knowledge"* [5]

Daniel J. Boorstin

We can send a person to the moon. We are capable of great accomplishments. Yet when it comes to the judgement of how much food we need to live, we are unable to figure it out by just looking at it. Why is that? It's because of the way our sight, brain and emotions work together.

After you eat a meal, you'll have no clue how many calories you just consumed unless you measured out and added up every ingredient first. Your brain does not have an indicator like a fuel gauge to let you know when you are full while you are eating. It takes at least 20 minutes for your brain to recognize that you have eaten enough. It's like filling up a gas tank without a mechanism to tell you you're about to overflow. Lots of gasoline would be spilled all over before you turned off the pump. Similarly, we usually overeat and respond to signs of overeating like: bloating, indigestion and other symptoms.

As intelligent as humans appear to be, we are unable to tell what is the right amount of food we need to eat. We make this decision with our eyes instead of our stomach. When we go to a restaurant, a portion is a plateful that is set in front of us. But the restaurant owner has a dilemma. When the cook prepares the food in the kitchen, they do not know who ordered it. Therefore, no matter who is sitting there, whether it's a five foot tall ballerina or a six foot tall football player, the cook has to prepare a portion big enough to satisfy either, so the portion is made for the football player.

Once the food arrives, we see that everyone's servings are just as big as ours. So it appears normal and we gulp it all down. We look around and see everyone eating the same amounts. We think we just ate one portion, yet we actually consumed two, three, four or more servings. Our brain just sees one portion.

Another problem with eating out is the fact that different consumers like different food types. One wants soup, another wants salad. Our generation is under the impression that we need a six course dinner for every meal. We look at a menu and see soup, salad, appetizer, entree, sides and a dessert, preferably paired with wine or soda. That's enough food to feed six Fatty-Buddies!

This is not just a problem in restaurants. Food is being sold in bigger containers and larger quantities everywhere, and people wrongly assume that a small package is a single serving. Next time you get what looks like an individual bottle of soda, peek at the label. The bottle probably contains two to three servings.

Oversized portions in restaurants are changing how we eat at home. We now expect the six course meal every day. We think that we need these huge portions. Our perceptions and our thoughts about food have changed. What is a portion size? What is the right portion size for you today vs. a year ago? Ten years ago? You need to know.

Unless we understand what it means, the serving size listed on a package is not always helpful to us as individuals. We are all different. We have different calorie needs, which depend on our size, age, gender, metabolism and physical activity. The USDA defines a serving size for many types of foods, and also tells us how much of each of the food groups we should eat. That's very helpful. But is a serving meant for the ballerina or the football player?

For example, when you glance at the nutrition facts of a package, you see that a serving has only 100 calories and three grams of fat. "That's not too bad," you think to yourself. What you did not notice was that the "serving size" was only one small cookie or 12 chips. Did you check to see whether the small, "individual" package actually contained three and a half servings? No, most of us listen to our brains. Our brain says, "You're not finished until the whole package is empty." Who really only eats one "serving" of snack food? Do you open a candy bar, take a bite and save the rest for later? Once you open the package you continue to eat until it's empty. There's no natural stopping point. Your brain does not have a gauge that tells you to stop filling. It says to take it all.

## CAUTION
**Some of the manufacturers, especially of candy bars, try to hide the calories by sealing the pack so that you have to unwrap part of it to find out the calories! Shame on them! Help stop this sneaky practice! Vote with your cash!**

We are living in an environment filled with information that we can't figure out, so we fall back on our senses to tell us when we have had enough. How full do you feel after you have a bowl of soup; do you still need a salad? Should you get a sandwich too? Oh, and can you find room for dessert? When and how do you decide to stop? When you are no longer hungry? When you feel satisfied? When you are stuffed? Or when you have cleaned your plate, no matter how much was there? Way too often, we choose the last one on that list.

We can't count on our senses! The food industry is constantly creating something new. We are presented with bigger and bigger portions. There are so many complex numbers thrown at us. Our brain "lies" to us and it's being constantly tricked. When it comes to the number of calories or the number of portions, how many are right for you today? How many will be right for you tomorrow? Should you have 200 calories for breakfast, 500 for lunch, and 1500 for dinner and 300 for snacks? Should you eat 300 calories every two hours instead?

How can you fight back? Who do you listen to? Who has the secret of how much food you and you alone need to eat to lose weight and to keep it off? Who can calculate for you how much you need today vs. tomorrow? There is only one person who can figure this out. It's you. Yes, you can do it without having a Ph.D. in math. All you need are the right tools for the job.

# Food for thought:

**Eureka:**    Our brain does not have a mechanism to tell us how many calories we have eaten.

**Note:**    A package is not a serving!

**Remember:**    There is a right portion size for you, for every stage of your life. This portion size will fluctuate depending on many factors. You can figure out what that size is and quickly adjust your dishware size to keep up with your pace of life.

**Beware:**    The extra food you eat today is the extra weight you will carry tomorrow.

# Chapter 5

# Your Eyes Lie

*"Perceive that which cannot be seen with the eye."* [6]
Miyamoto Musashi

When we were children, we saw the illusionists and magicians that performed tricks in front of our eyes. We believed in magic. As adults we know that these are just tricks our eyes play on us and the magic is gone. We may still be entertained, but we know that the secret to magic is in knowing how to do the trick.

We don't believe that we could be mislead by illusions, yet every day we are. Businesses are using marketing and advertising techniques to get us to purchase their products. They use illusion to get us to buy more and eat more food.

Our eyes can deceive us in many ways. They are not perfect in how they communicate with our brain. This is because of the relationship between our eyes and our brain. It has to do with the position of our eyes in relationship to each other and the delay in processing sight information.

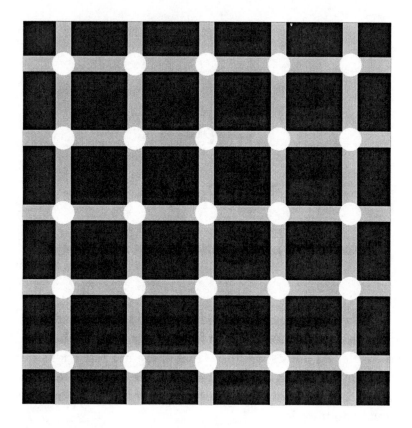

Because of this arrangement we are able to see depth and three dimensional objects and we can also be tricked by illusion. Look at each corner of the diagram above. As you move your eyes, do you notice small black dots flickering in the white circles? Your eyes will make you think that the small dots are bouncing from black to white.

A similar illusion occurs when you see the circles on the next page. As the black circles get bigger and bigger, the white circles appear to get smaller and smaller. That's right: they only appear smaller. In reality, they are not.

Every white circle is the exact same size. Now keep in mind the problem with our eyes and reality and let's shift gears back to eating.

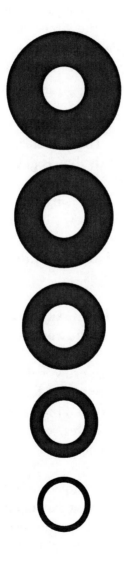

Over the last 20 to 30 years, dishes have been growing. A typical dinner plate used to be nine inches across; now it is 11 to 12 inches or more. What's wrong with the dishware getting bigger? What is wrong is that we did not realize that our food appeared smaller and smaller. The same illusion that you see with the white circles affects how we view our food. As our dishware was getting bigger and bigger we had to fill up our plates with more food just to feel like we were eating the same amount.

Plates were only the beginning of our problems. To match these beautiful, larger plates, all other eating-ware had to be enlarged. So the bowls got bigger, the spoons got bigger, and the forks, cups, glasses, etc. At the same time, restaurants were also increasing the size of their dishware. "Supersized" plates are now the norm everywhere. Our thoughts and perception of the right size food portion grew. Even our perception of what a healthy person looks like has been affected in our minds.

### The problem is, this supersized dishware made our food appear smaller!

So everything had to grow just to make us feel like we were eating the same amount. Restaurants increased the amount of food they served. Pizzas grew, bagels grew, bread slices grew, soda, chocolates, even fresh strawberries are bigger than they used to be.

The hardest part for us to admit is that we adults fell for this illusion. We were willing participants in this conspiracy. Unknowingly, we followed the newest trend like sheep. We set up our own traps and fell right into them.

There is a light at the end of the tunnel. **The illusion that got you to where you are today can get you back on the right path.** Your brain was tricked before and you can use the same trick in your favor. You just need to reverse the process. You can shrink your dishware slowly and gradually. The food will appear bigger and bigger. You will need less and less yet feel just as full. It works!

# If you don't do anything else as a result of reading this book, get smaller dishes!

How much smaller is the right dish size for me? Your basic dinner set typically has a dinner plate, a salad plate, and butter plate. That does not give you an option to slowly, in small increments, adjust your dishes. This is why we created our product which gives you the ability to do this gradually. You could try a different brand of dishware to get the in-between sizes. Every dish has a different style. Even though two dishes may look similar, they will have different food capacities. The slope of its sides and depth affect the amount of food contained. If you are not using pre-sized Dish Diet™ dishware to shrink the size of your dishware, check to ensure that you are actually changing your dish size in the right direction. Go to DishDiet.com℠ and verify your new dish size.

Start shrinking how you eat and you will shrink the amount of fat in your body. Your brain can be fooled a little at a time. But if you go too fast, your brain will know that you tricked it and it will punish you with a feeling of deprivation.

Start with your dishware. You'll get the quickest results. You then may need to shrink your glasses and cups, your snackware, your utensils and cutlery, etc. Starting with the dishware components that you use for foods that have the highest caloric density will give you the quickest results. For example:

- your ice cream dish
- your soda glass
- the spoon you use to serve gravy and dressing
- the dish you use for fried foods
- the dish you use for high cheese contents
- the dish you use for snacks

## THIS MAY BE THE BIGGEST STIMULUS TO YOUR BUDGET! SHRINKING YOUR DISHWARE WILL HELP EXPAND YOUR WALLET!

How much money would you save if you could cut your grocery bill in half or more? Depending how overweight you are, by shrinking the dishware and the amount of food you eat you will spend less and less on food.

Sorry Fatty-Buddy:

There is no room for your food on my new smaller plate!

# Food for thought:

*Illusion 1:*     Food appears smaller on a larger plate.

*Illusion 2:*     Food appears larger on a smaller plate.

*Fight:*          Fight illusion with illusion.

*Do:*             Change your dishware!

# Chapter 6

# Can A Plate Affect My Weight?

*"A pessimist sees the difficulty in every opportunity;
an optimist sees the opportunity
in every difficulty."* [7]

Winston Churchill

You still can't believe a dish can make you fatter? It can! Our parents and grandparents had dinner plates that were about nine inches in diameter. Today, plates are often over 12 inches wide. Some restaurants use 16-17 inch platters. As the plates got bigger, all eatingware and accessories had to grow to keep up with the plates.

On the next page, you see a single burger on a plate. Watch what happens to the burger as it is placed on the next larger size plate. See what happens when you put it on a platter? The burger appears to be shrinking. When you keep increasing the plate size, your brain believes there is less and less food. By the time it's on the big plate, the burger looks like a snack.

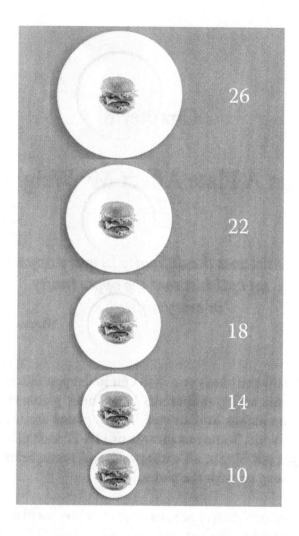

As the plates got bigger and bigger, the accessories on our tables got bigger, too. When the bowls got bigger, their capacity to deliver food grew even more than plates because of their shape. So even though the plates grew just a couple of inches in diameter, the bowls doubled in size. The glasses and mugs grew to keep up with the plates as well.

To keep up with the growing size of plates, we began putting more food on our plates than ever before. We are eating and drinking more, and are still feeling hungry. Our brains have learned to evaluate how much food we need by looking at our plate. But our brain can only tell how much empty space there is. Our eyes are deceived by the larger dishware and we think we need more food.

There was another phenomenon happening at the same time and we had no idea that it was affecting how much we eat. When you start eating on a bigger plate you reach for a bigger spoon and a bigger fork. Now, not only are you eating more food in every meal, you are eating more food in every bite. This means that you are transferring food from the plate to your mouth faster and faster.

Your utensils determine how fast the food is transferred into your mouth and down the hatch. Your brain has no idea how much food went down. For example, you eat a bowl of cereal with a teaspoon. You change the teaspoon size. Let's say the new teaspoon is twice as big as an old teaspoon. When you ate your cereal with the smaller teaspoon it took you 40 spoonfuls to finish your cereal. Now with the larger spoon it will only take 20 spoonfuls. Your brain doesn't care what spoon you used. All it knows is that you took only 20 spoonfuls and you used to get 40. Now you feel hungry!

When your cups and glasses get bigger, they impact your weight as well. If you just drank water it would not matter. But soda and juices, loaded with sugar and corn syrup, just add more pounds to your body without helping you feel satisfied. Let's say you always had a glass of soda with your meal. In the past a glass may have had 100 calories. Now "a glass" may hold 200 calories of the soda. You are drinking more calories without thinking about it.

When you have a big plate you will put more food on it. When you are drinking from a bigger glass, you will drink more calories. When you eat with bigger utensils, you will need more bites to keep you satisfied.

Some of today's cereal and soup bowls can hold a quart of liquid and even more solid food. When you put a 3/4 cup serving (typical recommended serving size on most cereal boxes) inside a quart size bowl, that bowl looks almost empty! With the new big spoons that will amount to two to three spoonfuls.

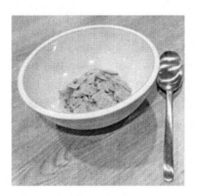 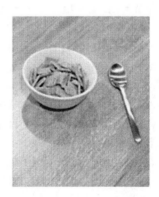

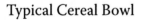

Typical Cereal Bowl            Dish Diet™ Bowl

So you justify pouring in four, five or more servings thinking "the serving size" is for children. You think, "That size portion can't really be for an adult!" You fill up your bowl. Well, you were wrong; the serving size **is** for an adult! That is all your body needs!

ALL the dishes and ALL our food portions along with them have exploded in size since the 1980's. The plates, the cups, the bowls, the snack bowls, the wine glasses, the burgers, the fries, the bagels... they all have been SUPERSIZED! As a result WE are becoming SUPERSIZED, too.

Can you believe that your dish has that much power over how much you eat? We pick up a plate or a bowl and start loading it up. When we look at our plate we are not looking to see how much food we piled on. We look at the "white space" that is still empty, and fill it up. (If you really want to see how poor our judgment is, go and watch people at a buffet.)

You can win the battle of the bulge, by using the dish/portion size that is right for you. Every one of us has a different metabolism. By monitoring your weight daily (same time of the day, preferably when you first wake up in the morning before you put your clothes on), you will learn how your body responds to the way you eat. You will see fluctuation, but you can respond to trends. When you see your weight going up or down too fast, you can respond by adjusting your dish/portion size with your next meal.

If you drop to the next smaller dish size, you may find that you are losing a pound or two a week. Typically that is OK for an adult, but check with your doctor to find out what is the best weight loss rate for you. If this rate of loss is acceptable, keep using the same size dish.

When you get to a weight level that's right for you, just stick to the size that helps you maintain that. You do not need to measure or count calories. You don't need to attend meetings or buy expensive foods. You eat your own food, your own way. When you gain weight, you simply shrink the size of your dishware. When you are maintaining your weight, stick to the same size as long as your lifestyle remains the same. If you find that you are losing too much weight, increase your dish/portion size. (But you already knew that.)

You will find that your diet is very similar from day to day. As long as your meals are the same size your body will get into a rhythm. The calories will average out. When you change your routine (for example, if you start eating more fried foods, or have less activity because you broke your leg), you will need to adjust your dish size.

What if your dish size got *so* small and you still are not losing weight? This can happen when your snacking habits have grown to the point that you are consuming too many calories. This could be as simple as a candy bar between meals, or a white chocolate mocha or a milkshake with your dinner. These may provide more calories than your body needs even if you do not eat much for breakfast, lunch or dinner.

Applying the Dish Diet™ program to your appetizers snacks, desserts and other foods with high CDM^SM (Caloric Density Mark^SM - see Chapter 14 for more information) will help you lose weight even faster. So you may want to measure the Dish Diet™ size of your snackware containers (check the DishDiet.com^SM website to determine the size) and reduce them gradually just like you would with your dishware.

Do not eat out of the package directly unless you know the exact size of the portion contained within the package.

So, what is so special about Dish Diet™ dishware? Every Dish Diet™ dish is sized using a new patent pending method. Just like you know your shirt size, you will get to know your portion size. The dishware sizes of plates and bowls correspond to each other. So if you are eating pasta on a size ten plate today and stew from a size ten bowl tomorrow, you are able to stick to your portion size. The plates and bowls can be used interchangeably as long as they are the same size.

Our vision is that every bowl or plate, every cup or glass, every spoon or fork and even pre-packaged food will be marked to help guide you and help you eat right every time. Keep checking the DishDiet.com℠ website, there's always something new "cooking" to help you succeed.

### CHANGE YOUR DISHWARE!

We know that this seems to be too easy! You probably think that we are trying to trick you. But what if it is that easy? What if this is the answer you've been waiting for? What do you have to lose by trying? Just your Fatty-Buddy!

*"This is one small step for [a] man,
one giant leap for mankind."*[7]

Neil Armstrong

# Food for thought:

*Size:*  The size of your dishware matters.

*Know:*  You need to know your portion or dishware size just like you know your shirt or your shoe size.

*Downsize:*  Shrink your dishware/portion size when you are gaining unwanted weight.

*Keep:*  Stick to your dishware/portion size to maintain healthy weight.

*Increase:*  Switch to the next larger dishware/portion size if you need to increase your weight.

*Adjust:*  Adjust your portion size up or down as your lifestyle and diet changes.

*Bigger:*  Bigger dishware results in more food served and more food eaten.

*Smaller:*  Smaller dishware will make you think you are eating more and result in you eating less.

# Chapter 7

# Change Doesn't Have To Be Hard

*"A man is but the product of his thoughts,
what he thinks, he becomes."*[8]

Mohandas Gandhi

So now that you know how the environment has changed, you need to act to change your environment. Although change may appear hard, it does not have to be. Research shows that we may not even detect small changes in daily calorie intake if the adjustments are only 100 to 200 calories. Compare this small change to the changes in your life caused by living with obesity. The changes discussed in this book will be a piece of cake (pardon the comparison) compared to a life with diabetes or after a stroke. Here is the Dish Diet℠ motto:

## Eat Less - Move More

Sound too easy? Well, it can be easy if you make these changes in small, gradual steps.

**Change your dishware.** The size of your dishware is important. If you use the Dish Diet$^{SM}$ you will find that it will not be any harder to go from size 25 to 24 than from 16 to 15. The patent pending formula for Dish Diet$^{SM}$ sizes adjusts automatically with every size.

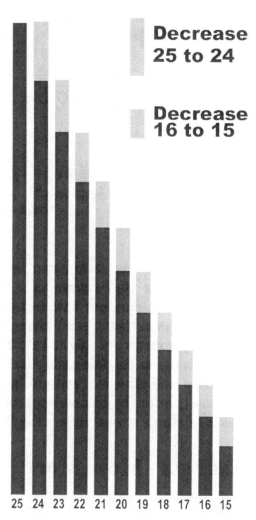

**Decrease 25 to 24**

**Decrease 16 to 15**

25 24 23 22 21 20 19 18 17 16 15

Even though you reduce your dish size by 1 size, the reduction in food portion changes as the sizes decrease to keep you motivated! This is true regardless of what your typical diet is.

For example, let's say Jack and Jill are going on a diet together. Jack's starting dish size is 25 and Jill's starting dish size is 18. They both reduce their dish size by 1 size, Jack to 24 and Jill to 17 . The Jack's portion will shrink by more calories than Jill's because her starting size is smaller. When they are ready to reduce their size even further, they can both go down together by one size. Now Jack shifts to Dish Diet™ size 23 and Jill to size 16. Even though Jack will again reduce the amount of calories he consumes, the calorie reduction between size 24 and 23 is smaller than the calorie reduction between size 25 and 24. This is true for Jill as well; the reduction from size 17 to 16 is smaller than going from size 18 to 17. The decrease in calories between sizes keeps shrinking as the sizes get smaller and shifting to a smaller size gets easier and easier. This is what helps you stay motivated.

The Dish Diet™ sizes take into account the changes in our Basal Metabolic Rate (see Chapter 13) as we lose weight and allow you to customize you dish/portion size.

**Change how you select your dishware.** Would you buy clothes without first looking at what size they are? No, yet you are using dishware that affects how much you eat without knowing its size. The reason you do it is because until now, there was no way of knowing how big dishware is. As your dishware shrinks in size, so will your clothing size. KNOW YOUR DISH SIZE!

**Change how you serve yourself.** When you eat at home, serve yourself in the kitchen and put the leftovers away immediately. Do not put serving dishes on the table. We no longer listen to our bodies when it comes to feeling full. Once you taste your first bite, it's difficult to stop eating. Temptation is hard to fight.

Give yourself a chance to succeed by making it hard to get that second helping. Use logic before emotion kicks in. SERVE and HIDE.

**Change how you select your food.** All food has calories, but not all food will make you feel as full for longer periods of time. For example, nutritionists recommend eating high fiber foods to help you feel more satisfied even though visually the portions may be the same size.

All foods vary in their caloric density, which is the number of calories in a given volume. You can eat everything you like, but if you eat foods that have high caloric density you will consume more calories per portion. You can reduce your calorie consumption gradually by changing what you put on your dish. Start by replacing one spoonful of food that has high caloric density with food that has lower caloric density. You will learn more about caloric density later on in this book. GRADUALLY TRANSITION TO FOODS WITH LOWER CALORIC DENSITY.

**Change how you eat your food.** Until now we paid very little attention to how we ate. The authors have developed a way to size the utensils that transfer the food to your mouth. The faster you "shovel" it in, the faster you will eat your meal and your brain will not even register that you ate something.

The bigger your spoon and your fork, the faster you will transfer the food to your mouth. The more food in each mouthful, the less opportunity you'll have to taste it. Because a lot of this food will not even come into contact with your taste receptors, it will be transferred to your stomach without being registered as received. Using smaller utensils with smaller Bite Size$^{SM}$ will help you control how fast you transfer the food to your mouth and give you an opportunity to swish it around so you can taste every flavor. You will eat slower, feel fuller and eat less. SHRINK YOUR BITE SIZE$^{SM}$.

**Change how you eat in a restaurant.** Today we are eating out more than we used to. Restaurants are competing for our business. They want you to come back, so they give you bigger dishes, 4-6 course meals, huge desserts. Everyone gets served the same size meal, whether you need it or not. Use the same size dish as you use at home, ask for a box and pack the rest away to take home before you start eating.

Making the decision of what you're going to eat before you taste the food is a lot easier. Once the food is packed away and out of sight, you are not going to have "just one more bite." Chances are that by the time you get home, your stomach and your brain will both be satisfied.

You may not be comfortable doing this if you go out with your friends, "What will they think?" Well, if they are truly your friends, they will support you wholeheartedly.

Order one course at a time. It will mean more work for the waiter and the kitchen. If they do not like it they will change their ways. IT'S YOUR MONEY!

**Change your environment.** The surroundings and how you live affect how much you eat. It will be harder for you to lose weight when the whole world around you reminds you of food. Having snacks nearby and handy does not build your character or the strength of your will. But it sure is a way to ensure that Fatty-Buddy does not get hungry.

We typically think about food throughout a day! If you add external influences to your environment, you will think about food approximately 200 times per day. [9]

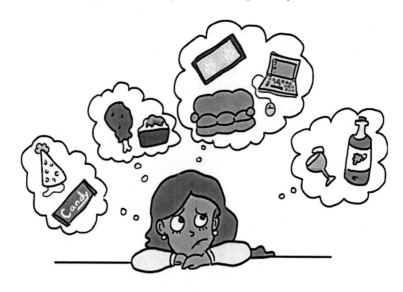

You can't eliminate your thoughts, but you can use the same strategy to make you think about food less often and healthy activities more.

Look at your surroundings where you work, where you live, where you spend your leisure time. Are there any "food-thought" triggers? How much time do you spend in your kitchen? Every time you look up, you see the refrigerator and your pantry. Fight marketing with marketing. You need to design a marketing campaign that's right for you. What will make you think about walking, dancing or playing sports? These are the visual reminders you need to surround yourself with.

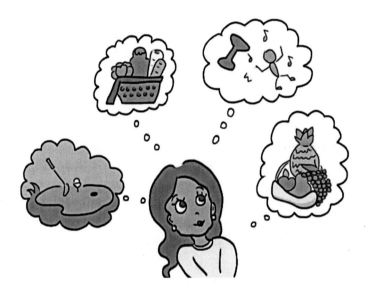

Here are some examples of how you can counter the environment's marketing:

- Where your candy jar stood before, put a weight for training and lifting while you have a free moment.

- Hide your cookbooks from the counter top and put nice photos of delicious fresh vegetables.

- Don't buy and store foods you crave!

- Replace what triggers your thoughts of food with thoughts of activity.

- Hide your vices from your eyes.

- Record TV, then fast forward through commercials.

Marketing techniques work. You just need to use them yourself to counteract your environment. You can help your brain to think about fun and exercise. You can market to your brain the healthier foods. You can retrain your brain to eat the right portion size for you. MARKETING WORKS!

**Change how much you move.** Adding exercise to our already full, stressful day seems impossible. But adding more movement gradually can be simple. When we are overweight, it is harder to move. As we lose weight, it will get easier and easier. Start shifting in increments to the activities that will burn more calories and do a little more of each.

Many of us try to lose weight by adding exercise to our routine. What we do not realize is that as we lose weight we will burn fewer calories for the same amount of effort. For example, a 300 pound person will burn 576 calories running for 30 minutes at 5 mph (running 2.5 miles in 30 minutes). But as we lose more and more weight, we will burn fewer and fewer calories doing the same activity.

### Weight in Pounds vs. Calories Burned [10]

| Weight | 300 | 280 | 260 | 240 | 220 | 200 | 180 | 160 | 140 | 120 |
|---|---|---|---|---|---|---|---|---|---|---|
| Calories | 576 | 538 | 499 | 461 | 422 | 384 | 346 | 307 | 269 | 230 |

We get demotivated. That's why it's important to keep increasing the amount of activity while reducing the portion size at the same time. Doing this gradually in small increments will be the most successful in the long run.

So for every reduction of your dish/portion size, increase your amount of activity in 2-5 minute increments. As you weigh less and less, this will get easier and easier. In 30 weeks you can go from walking 1 minute a day to 30 minutes a day by just adding 1 minute a week. You will not feel that increase and it will keep getting easier and easier.

You can increase the amount of activity in your daily routine by making small changes. Here is an example of the number of calories you will burn in 60 minutes of an activity if you weigh 150 lbs.

**Calories Burned in 60 Minutes
by a Person Weighing 150 Pounds** [11]

| Activity | Sleep | Sit | Stand | Walk 2 mph | Aerobic Dance | Jog 6 mph |
|---|---|---|---|---|---|---|
| Calories Burned | 90 | 114 | 150 | 198 | 546 | 654 |

So if you spend a lot of time in bed doing things, get up and sit. If you do a lot of your activities sitting, stand up as much as you can. If you are standing, can you walk? If you walk, can you run?

You can dance while you are cooking, cleaning, getting dressed, doing laundry and watching TV. Take a look at your current lifestyle. Find where you can add more movement a little bit at a time. Put weights in front of your snacks. Before you open a bag of snacks, lift the weights for as long as needed to burn the calories you plan to eat. DANCE! WALK! RUN!

**Reminder: Consult your medical professional before adding exercise, even in small increments.**

**Change how you shop. Never go to the store hungry.** Eat before shopping for food. You will not buy as much. Reorganize your shopping list the way you want to go through the store. Don't even head down the snack aisle. Go through the non-food isles first. Fill up your cart with products like paper towels, detergent and coffee. Then go through the fresh fruit and vegetable aisle. Even the shopping carts are bigger than they used to be! Fill them up with good foods; you will have less room for junk food. SHOP SMARTER!

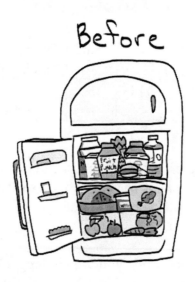

Before

**Change how you store food.** Keeping foods that you crave out of sight is going to help you with your marketing strategy. If you have to have foods you crave at home, keep them out of sight and out of reach. Put them in closed containers that you can't see through. Put healthier foods with lower Caloric Density Mark$^{SM}$ in places that are easier to reach. DON'T BUY JUNK, but if you do, HIDE JUNK FOODS OUT OF SIGHT!

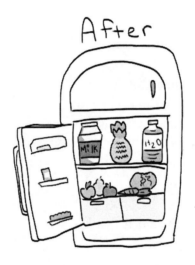

You can help change our environment. You have the powerful tool that can change the government, as well as the food and restaurant industries.

### YOU HAVE THE POWER OF THE DOLLAR!

Every dollar you spend on bad foods will create more demand for those bad foods. Use the power of your money to make a change for you, your family and the future generations.

# What has changed?

**Bigger:**
- dishes
- drinkware
- pantries
- refrigerators
- restaurant portions

**More:**
- sugar added
- salads with high calorie dressings
- eating out
- cheese added to many foods
- watching TV (TV set in every room)
- exposure to food commercials (TV, internet, billboards)
- additional freezers
- high calorie condiments
- alcohol with dinner
- fast food
- coffee houses (high calorie drinks)
- deep fried foods
- "bad food" advertised everywhere
- social activities combined with food
- snack machines
- soda, juices and high calorie drinks
- alcohol with every social gathering
- exciting packaging with high quality photos
- sedentary relaxation activities due to exhaustion
- buying in big quantities
- processed foods (last longer than fresh foods)

**Less:**
- time (fresh food requires shopping more often)
- activity (drive everywhere, internet, video games)
- time for food preparation  (both parents working)
- fresh fruit/vegetables (go bad faster)
- time spent outdoors (air conditioning, kid safety)

**Other Changes:**
- restaurants serve limited fruit/vegetables
- family rooms open to the kitchens (one space)
- "bad foods" more flavorful

# Food for thought:

*Change:*      your dishware.

*Change:*      how you serve yourself.

*Change:*      how you select foods.

*Change:*      how you transfer your food to your mouth.

*Change:*      how you eat at home and in restaurants.

*Change:*      your environment.

*Change:*      how much you move.

*Change:*      how you shop.

*Change:*      how you store food.

# Part 2:

# The Present - Action

# Chapter 8

# How Does The Dish Diet<sup>SM</sup> Work?

*"A person with a new idea is a crank until the idea succeeds."* [12]

Mark Twain

Just as technology is changing at rapid rates, we saw a need for changing how we eat and how we live. The old tools do not work in the new, ever-changing environment. We looked at the trends and envisioned where we are heading if we stay on the current path.

We have examined the process of eating. We believe that how we eat makes a great difference in how much we eat. As a result we have invented a program called Dish Diet<sup>SM</sup>, a new patent pending way of eating. Although most of us view diet as a deprivation of food, Dish Diet<sup>SM</sup> aims to take this word back to its original meaning of "the foods eaten".

Dish Diet<sup>SM</sup> does not stop you from eating any particular foods - quite the opposite. We encourage you to eat a well balanced diet. Our bodies need a variety of foods to provide the nutrients necessary to maintain good health. You will, however, be able to reduce the amount of food you eat. Just remember, to lose weight, you must burn up more calories than you consume or eat fewer calories than you burn. Although physical activity is important for good health, it is much easier to avoid eating those extra 100 calories than it is to run long enough to burn them off. As you follow this program, you will gradually get used to eating less. YOU decide how fast you want to lose weight. You also will have a set of dishware that will help you take the first steps, and make it easy to change how you view the word "diet."

When do you find yourself thinking about food? Is it a time of the day? Are you eating because you thought of food or because someone else has mentioned it? What's the size of your dishware? Do you go out to eat? Do you eat while you cook? Are you the type of person who shops on the way home from work when you are famished?

Researchers at Cornell University determined that we make more than 200 food-related decisions per day.[13] That's one thought every five minutes. Your dishes, the environment, your friends and the impact of being on a deprivation diet, are all causing you to think about food constantly. Some of us are making plans for what we will have for lunch when we are eating our breakfast. Those of us that do the food shopping, planning and cooking for the week spend even more time thinking about food.

Some diets require you to plan your meals and calculate what you're going to eat for every part of the day. This causes you to think about food throughout the day. When you use

Dish Diet™ dishware, all you need to know is your dish size. By using the same size throughout the day, you will get into the rhythm of life. You will eliminate the constant calculating and planning.

If you need to refuel every three to four hours, just pick the dish that's your size and fill it up. You will not need to think about how many calories are in the chicken, or the potato, or the broccoli or the carrots. You will just fill and eat. The number of calories may vary per meal just like the amount of activity you will do from day to day. Some days you will eat more and other days you will eat less. But in the long run, as long as you consume food using the same dish/portion size, your daily amount will average out.

With Dish Diet™ you are not controlling every ingredient that you consume. You are controlling the average daily consumption without thinking about food. You will automate how you eat, and how you eat impacts how much you eat. If you could measure every crumb of food and control every calorie you burn your day might look like this:

| EAT | BURN | RESULT |
| --- | --- | --- |
| 1000 calories | 1000 calories | No weight change |
| 1100 calories | 1000 calories | Store 100 calories and GAIN 10 pounds/year |
| 900 calories | 1000 calories | Remove 100 calories from "storage" and lose 10 pounds/year! |

Every day you don't burn all the calories you eat, they go in your "trunk". You put a little more fat around your waist and on your thighs. The difference between cars and our bodies is that our skin stretches like a balloon so we can store more and more. But our organs are designed to carry a certain load. So when we overload our body, eventually it breaks down.

You know you should eat less, so you decide to start some "diet." Most "diets" begin with a sudden, drastic cut in calories. You know what that means. You get hungry and cranky. You feel deprived. You think about food all of the time. What you may not know is that your body reacts as if you were actually starving. Your metabolism slows down to conserve the energy. This makes it even harder to lose weight!

The Dish Diet<sup>SM</sup> is different. It works with your body and brain to help you succeed. It helps you eat fewer calories over time without suddenly starving yourself. Research shows that you can easily eat 100 to 200 calories more or less each day without your body noticing. [13] With Dish Diet<sup>SM</sup> you will lower your average daily calorie consumption a little at a time.

How are you supposed to control your portion size if you don't know what your portion size is? How do you control something that you don't measure? How do you control something that is constantly changing?

There is no meter that you can plug into your body that will tell you "Today you will need 1500 calories" or as the day goes on "You ate 400 calories so far today. You have 1100 left for the rest of the day! This meal is 1800 calories; you will overeat! You will feel pain and suffer through the night, guaranteed." There is no easy way to calculate all that. Yet the government and latest research tells us to control our portion. What does that mean?

You could measure every ingredient in your food and add it up to keep track of every bite and calorie you take in. You could plan out your calories for the day. For example, let's assume you need approximately 1500 calories per day, then your day may look like this:

| Breakfast: | 200 | Snack: | 100 |
|---|---|---|---|
| Snack: | 100 | Dinner: | 600 |
| Lunch: | 400 | Snack: | 100 |

Then you will need to weigh and measure every ingredient that goes into the meal. You will have to make sure to eat 200 calories for breakfast. If you eat 250 instead you will need to reduce some other meal by 50 calories later in the day.

Those who tried this type of diet know how hard it is to do the math every time you open your mouth to eat. You end up readjusting your plan throughout the day each time you eat more than allowed (very seldom will you eat less.) Not only is this time consuming, it also will greatly increase the amount of time you spend thinking about food. Is that how you want to live?

Limiting calories will make you feel deprived and at some point, like so many of us in the past, you will give up. There is a better way. A way that you can eat comfort food without worrying how many calories it contains. You do not need to walk around with a calculator all day long. You will not have to look up the slice of pizza in your calorie log and measure it to see if it has 200 or 400 calories. You will find that you think less about food and more about living.

Why is Dish Diet<sup>SM</sup> different? As inventors we have an engineering mindset. We look at eating as a complete system. A system that involves not just the food. A system that is made up of many individual processes of how we decide, select, prepare, serve and consume food.

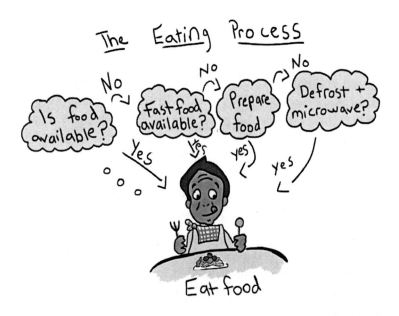

There are many decision points throughout this process, and at each point our decisions can be influenced by factors that have absolutely nothing to do with hunger or your body's actual needs. We believe this is why we are getting bigger and bigger. This problem has exploded in the past 20-30 years. The human race has not changed, yet our environment has changed and keeps changing at an incredible rate.

As engineers, we look at an eating process that is made up of many steps:

- Something triggers a thought about food: time of day, someone else is eating, smell something, another thought reminds you of the dinner last night, pass a vending machine or fast food place...

- If the food is right there we will probably not even think about it but pop it in our mouth.

- We might even go through a logical self determination to justify eating. For example, it might go something like this: "Oh, Jack brought doughnuts! Should I have one? I just had breakfast an hour ago. Maybe I should wait, but if I wait they will all be gone. All right, I will take one and save it for later, but it will not taste as good as it would now. OK, I'll have half now and half later. No, the other half will dry out...Wow, that went quick! Maybe I should have another..."

- We then decide what we feel like eating. For example, is it a one course or a multi-course meal. We ask ourselves "How hungry do I feel? Am I just a little hungry or am I famished?"

- We select the location where to get food.

- We prepare or buy food.

- We select the dishware we will use.

- We select the utensils we will use.

- We serve ourselves.

- We select drinkware and the type of drink.

- We eat while focusing on food, or TV, or conversation.

- We finish what we served and decide whether we want more. If so, we get seconds or even thirds.

- We then decide whether we feel like something sweet. If so, what will satisfy our sweet palate?

There are many other steps depending on what type of meal you are going to eat. The point is that most diets concern themselves with food itself, yet all these other steps are very critical in how much food you will consume.

The Dish Diet[SM] automates some of these steps so that you do not have to think how many calories you need to save for dinner. We are all creatures of habit. Even though our daily meals may differ every day, we will consume the same amount on the average. What Dish Diet[SM] tries to accomplish is to make your eyes happy. Users of the program will automate their eating so that all the person needs to know is their dish or portion size and follow it for all meals and snacks. This helps the body to get into rhythm of fuel (eat) then burn and keeps the metabolism at a higher rate than sudden drastic caloric reduction.

The timing of your meals will depend on your comfort level, and your ability to get time to eat in your daily schedule. Some of you may be able to eat every four hours and as portions get smaller, shorter intervals may be necessary. This may require you to have more smaller meals per day.

When you select your clothes or shoes  you don't just pick "one-size-fits-all". So why are you eating from dishware that is "one-size-fits-all - BIG!" The question is what is your dish/portion size today? You can go to DishDiet.com™ to find out your size. DishDiet™ dishware makes it easy for you to know what size your dish/portion is. Once you know your size, you change your dishware, gradually adjusting to the next size down to reduce your weight. You can increase the size to help increase your weight. To maintain your weight you adjust the size up or down as necessary.

## WHAT'S YOUR DISH SIZE?

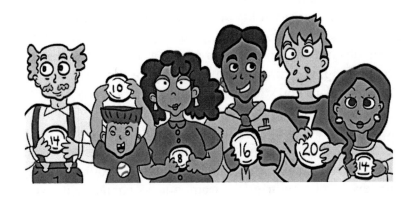

With Dish Diet™, as your dish size gradually gets smaller, you can fit less food on it, yet it's always full. Reducing the dish size in small increments will not make you feel deprived. Your dish will get a little smaller, but remember the illusion we discovered. The same amount of food will appear a little bigger. You will fill up your plate with less food, but you will feel like you're eating same amount as before. You end up eating less yet feel satisfied. The steps are small and the food still fills the plate, so you don't really notice the difference.

One of the questions we often get is, "What's to stop me from going for a second or a third smaller plate?" Our answer is "You!" You are the only person who is able to do this. Chances are that those who asked already are going for the second and third plate. The beauty of Dish Diet$^{SM}$ is that when you gradually shrink your dishware you will gradually shrink all helpings!

If you weigh yourself every morning before breakfast, you will learn how your body responds to the new dish/portion size with every size change. This weight will fluctuate depending how late you ate the night before, the amount of water you are retaining and other factors of your metabolism. You will learn how much your weight goes up and down normally and whether you are seeing a trend. If the trend is creeping up, you downsize. If it's going in the direction you are happy with you stick to the size.

Many guides suggest that you use the size of your fist to determine your portion size. Think about it, the size of your fist does not change that much throughout your adult life. However, your calorie requirements do change with your age and your lifestyle changes. What do you think will be the reaction of a person, who is currently consuming 10 fistfuls, when you tell them that they need to limit their portion to one fistful? Don't measure your portion with your wrist, use the size of your dish.

Unlike other diets Dish Diet<sup>SM</sup> enables you go at your own unique pace. You don't have to focus on measuring or counting points or calories. You don't have to eat expensive, tasteless, pre-packaged foods. You don't have to attend meetings. You can lose weight as quickly or as slowly as you want, just by changing your dish size. Dish Diet<sup>SM</sup> puts YOU in control!

# Food for thought:

*Change:*    Change how you eat, not what you eat.

*Adjust:*    Adjust your portion size with the dish size to maintain weight.

*Small:*    Adjusting in small increments will help you succeed.

*Your food:*    Eating food that you like and adjusting the amounts in small increments will help change your brain's perception and teach you how to eat to stay healthy.

# Chapter 9

# How Do I Start?

*"A man may die, nations may rise and fall,
but an idea lives on."*[19]

John F. Kennedy

Starting a Dish Diet℠ program is easy. You do not need to purchase the set of dishes. You can put a nail in a wall with a brick yet a hammer makes it easier. You can try to implement the Dish Diet℠ yourself but the Dish Diet™ Dishware makes it easier. The dishware comes pre-sized with our unique formula that allows you to use a plate or bowl of the same size in order to stick to your program.

To use a set of Dish Diet℠ dishes you would:

1. Pick a plate.
2. Check your weight.
3. Feel great.
4. Change the plate to lose more weight.

Use your new Dish Diet™ dishes for all your meals and snacks. Hiding your old dishes out of sight will help you succeed. (Removing temptation from your sight and from easy reach will be an easy step that you can take to help you lose weight.)

PLEASE CHECK WITH YOUR DOCTOR BEFORE STARTING ANY NEW DIET OR WEIGHT LOSS PLAN!

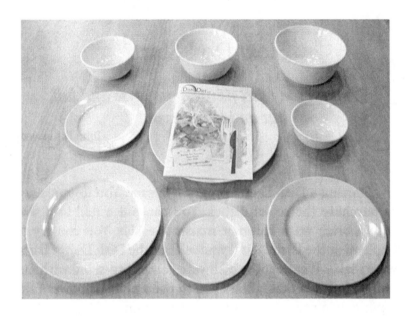

The Dish Diet™ dishware is made of high quality porcelain. The dishes look and feel like typical eating-ware. The Dish Diet™ dishware has an established food capacity that is represented by a single number. Each plate and bowl is assigned a unique Dish Diet™ Size that you can use to help guide you during this life-changing process. The current set consists of five plates and four bowls. Each item has the Dish Diet™ size imprinted on the back. The current set has the numbers decreasing in increments of five. This appears to be effective for most users.

If you still find it too difficult to transition from one size to the next we may be able to provide you with a single dish of another size. You can contact DishDiet.com<sup>SM</sup> to get more information.

To start your Dish Diet<sup>SM</sup> journey, you first choose a starting size. Put your food on the dish you normally use. Then, transfer that food to a Dish Diet<sup>TM</sup> dish that will just fit all of it. That's your starting Dish size. Do the same for a meal for which you use a bowl.

For example, take out your current cereal bowl. Put in the cereal you'd normally eat. Transfer the cereal to a Dish Diet<sup>TM</sup> Bowl that just fits your cereal. That is your starting bowl. It may be that you can't fit all of the food onto any of the Dish Diet<sup>TM</sup> dishes. That's OK. Just start with the largest size.

Some of us tend to overfill the dish more than usual when we first start, since we have the old feeling of "I'm on a deprivation diet" and panic. So simply try a dish, and if it does not do what you want it to do, change to a smaller or bigger size. It's that simple.

### DIRECTIONS (FOR ADULTS ONLY)

Weigh yourself every day, at the same time each day. We recommend each morning before breakfast and before you get dressed, so that your weight is not affected by any food you may have just consumed or clothing you wear that day. After a week of using the Dish Diet℠ dishes for all your meals, check if your weight is changing.

To decide what to do the next week, follow the directions below unless your doctor gives you other guidelines. If at any time you have questions, contact us through DishDiet.com℠ website.

If you:

## Lost 3 or more pounds

The plate/bowl is too small. You should change to the next larger size dish. Most doctors recommend maximum weight loss of 2 pounds per week for an adult.

## Lost 1-2 pounds

Great, that's a typically recommended rate for adult weight loss. Are you feeling OK? If everything is going well, continue using the same size plate and bowl.

## Stayed the same

Then you are still eating too much. Shrink your plate and bowl to the next smaller size.

## Gained weight

OOPS! Yes, it can happen. Sometimes we can't help but be aware of the change, and unconsciously pile on more food or started to eat foods that were on your forbidden list. Don't worry, just shrink your dish size to the next smaller size.

The SECRET is to use the dish/portion size to control your weight. To lose weight, use a smaller size dish. To gain weight, use a bigger size dish. How fast you lose weight is up to you. Slow and steady is healthier and easier, since it maximizes your metabolic rate!

You are in control! You can even use the Dish Diet$^{SM}$ dishes to maintain a healthy weight throughout your life – just find the size that's right for you.

## WATCH YOUR PLATE - LOSE THE WEIGHT!

If you are not ready to purchase the dishes, that's OK. You can still start the Dish Diet$^{SM}$ program. Although, it will be harder for you to know what plate and bowl are equivalent to each other. The other issue is finding nice porcelain dishes that shrink incrementally at Dish Diet$^{TM}$ size intervals.

Every style of plate or bowl, while it may appear the same size, is different. They all vary in the amount of food they can hold. So unknowingly you might select a dish that looks smaller but it actually could hold more food.

That's why the sizing is so important. It ensures that when you downsize you really are downsizing. So if you do want to use your own dishware, be sure to check its Dish Diet$^{TM}$ size on our website first.

No matter what, you can still get started. Start with your own dish and look for a similar dish that is just a little smaller. Check its Dish Diet$^{TM}$ size. Keep using that dish for a week. If you are losing too quickly or gaining you may not want to wait a week. You monitor your weight and follow directions above.

## You will be amazed how little food you truly need to refuel!

Dish Diet[SM] program goes to the roots of what diet truly means. Dish Diet[SM] program is a new revolutionary way of eating and simplified healthier living. Here are examples of how you could use it for the rest of your life:

Your doctor just told you that you need to lose 30 pounds or else you are at high risk for some serious problem. First you go to DishDiet.com[SM]. You either purchase a starter set or you find out the size of your current dishware. Let's say that your current dish size is 28. Then this is the dish size that got you to be 30 ponds heavier than you need to be to stay healthy. So now you get a dish size 27. Chances are that you eat a variety of foods so you may need to find the dish size of your plate and your bowl and adjust both by one size. You would check your weight daily while using the smaller dish size. By end of the week , how did you do?

You find that you lost two pounds. Well since your goal is to lose weight and you are an adult, your doctor might feel that this is great. The following week you find that you did not lose any weight. So you would change your bowl and your plate to size 26. The following week you lost another two pounds, you keep the same size. The following week you have not lost any weight. Time to go to plate size 25 and so on. Once you reach your goal weight, let's say dish size 15, you can stick to your dish size to maintain it as long as your lifestyle remains unchanged.

After you are at your weight goal you decide that not only do you want to lose weight, but you also want to improve your diet. Instead of eating fried chicken every day you will fill half of your dish with vegetables. Well now you might find that you are losing too much weight, what do you do? Increase your dish size and maybe you can now use dish size 18. A year later you break a leg, you cannot exercise and now you started to gain weight again, so you downsize your dish/portion size to size 16. And so on...

Note: The Dish Diet™ dishware starter set includes five plates and four bowls. We selected the sizes that work for most users. (A complete set would contain 60 items, which is not necessary for most people.)

Not only can you lose weight with the Dish Diet℠ program, but you can prevent the excess gain to start with. You can maintain a healthy weight simply by adjusting your Dish Diet℠ size as needed when you start gaining weight. The table below shows what a portion/dish size may look like over your life span. As we grow from childhood to adulthood, our portion size gradually increases. When we reach our twenties and thirties we max out and then gradually as we get older, we need fewer and fewer calories since our bodies burn less.

# The Dish Diet: Watch Your Plate Not Your Weight

| Age | Women Daily Calories | | Men Daily Calories | |
|---|---|---|---|---|
| 0-5 | | 1000 | | 1000 |
| 5-10 | | 1200 | | 1400 |
| 10-15 | | 1600 | | 1800 |
| 15-20 | | 1800 | | 2200 |
| 20-25 | | 2000 | | 2400 |
| 25-30 | | 2000 | | 2400 |
| 30-35 | | 1800 | | 2200 |
| 35-40 | | 1800 | | 2200 |
| 40-45 | | 1800 | | 2200 |
| 45-50 | | 1800 | | 2200 |
| 50-55 | | 1600 | | 2000 |
| 55-60+ | | 1600 | | 2000 |

Note: The age ranges in table above are shown for sedentary levels of activity and they have been slightly shifted to help demonstrate the concept. See Appendix 2 for original age ranges.[15]

Unfortunately, we continue to eat like we are in our twenties and have a difficult time shrinking our portion size even though our bodies do not need as much food. Now Dish Diet[SM] gives you the flexibility you need. You can make small adjustments periodically and maintain your healthy way of living. You are finally able to act even preventively when you know what your plans are. Here are some examples:

| Life Change | Dish/Portion Size Adjustment |
|---|---|
| Moved South-eat more fried food | Downsize |
| Moved to California- eat more lower caloric density foods | Increase size |
| Break a leg- limited mobility | Downsize |
| Summer-running outside | Increase size |
| Winter-can't run outside | Downsize |
| Going on cruise- more food availability | Downsize |
| Joined gym- actually using it | Increase size |
| Holidays-more food availability and temptation | Downsize |

The greatest benefit is that you can lose weight while eating the foods you love. You do not need to buy expensive diet foods. There is nothing special or magical about these foods. They use the same ingredients that you use. The only difference is that they measure it for you, and package it in a box with a delicious looking label. When you open the package and heat it up, it doesn't look as good as the label, does it? Next you will transfer your food to your regular dish and you see how it shrinks even more.

With Dish Diet™ you can eat delicious foods that are freshly made and haven't been frozen for months. You do not deprive yourself of any type of food. Once you learn how to shrink your  thoughts about food, you will be ready to hear how to make your diet healthier. Adding foods that have lower caloric food densities will help you keep a bigger dish size and maintain your weight or help you loose weight faster without the feeling of deprivation.

# Food for thought:

**Lose:**       Lose weight by adjusting your dish/size gradually at your own pace.

**Gain:**       Gain confidence that you can control your weight.

**Easy:**       Losing weight can be easy when you have the right tools.

**Tools:**       Your tools are in your cabinets. Finding out their Dish Diet$^{SM}$ size is a lot easier than measuring how many calories every ingredient is in your meal.

**Change:**       Change how you eat so you can change how you live.

# Chapter 10

# Small Changes Lead To Big Success

*"Be faithful in small things because it is in them that your strength lies."* [16]

Mother Teresa

The Dish Diet[SM.] is all about making small, gradual changes. Working with your mind and your body to succeed. You gradually get used to eating smaller and smaller amounts of food without feeling deprived.

For example, today you may be eating 50 candies as a snack. Well if tomorrow you start to eat 45, will you feel deprived? No, but if you cut down to 25 or stop eating them altogether you probably would. So for next week, try to eat only 45, and the following week 40, and so on. In a few months you will have lost weight, and will be satisfied with only a few for a snack.

That's the same principle the Dish Diet[SM] program follows. Small gradual changes can result in big sustainable successes.

Some of us are impatient and want to lose weight FAST. You can do that with Dish Diet[SM.] because you are in control. But most doctors recommend a slower rate of one to two pounds a week maximum. This is healthier, keeps your metabolism high, and is more likely to result in permanent changes. Chances are, you did not gain all that weight in six weeks, and you shouldn't try to lose it that fast either.

You are not just trying to lose weight, you are also retraining your brain and your body to eat right and live well. It takes time, so be patient with yourself. Give yourself a chance to succeed.

According to research by Brian Wansink, "by making 100-200 calorie changes in your daily intake you won't feel deprived and backslide."[17] You will be rewarded with a 10 to 20 pounds weight loss in one year!

This concept can be applied to other habits too, not just food. For example: physical activity. Begin walking five minutes each day. After a week, walk for seven or eight minutes every day. Increase at your own rate, and eventually you will be getting the recommended 30 minutes of activity most days. Remember, a gradual change is much easier accomplish and to sustain over a long period of time.

The current Dish Diet™ dishware set has five plates, sized in increments of "5". With every five sizes you drop, add five minutes to your exercise routine. As you lose more and more weight your exercise will become easier and easier. If you increase your exercise by five minutes every time you drop in a dish size, after six weeks you will be up to 30 minutes per day.

A reminder: *You need to check with your doctor before you start a new exercise regime or increase your exercise.*

Remember how we've said that the Dish Diet<sup>SM</sup> program will change how you eat? Well not only do you need to change the size of your bowls and your plates, you need to change all your dishware SLOWLY AND GRADUALLY. Dish Diet<sup>SM</sup> sizing system works for your drinkware and your utensils. You can go to DishDiet.com<sup>SM</sup> and find out the current Dish Diet<sup>SM</sup> size of your cups and glasses. Gradually shrinking the drinkware that you use for your high caloric density drinks like soda, alcohol and milkshakes will help you optimize your weight. Increasing the size of the drinkware that you use for water or green tea, for example, will help you get more of these into your life.

**Why is changing your drink-ware so important?** It's because our environment has added a lot of high caloric density foods that come in liquid form. A milkshake is a huge meal by itself, not an addition to a meal. A large White Chocolate Shake by White Castle™ in the Cincinnati area is 1330 calories; for some of us that is the total number of calories we should eat all day, not an addition to a meal!

When we said we are revolutionizing how we eat, we meant every aspect of eating. Your utensils are just as important in changing how you eat as your dishware. We have introduced the concept of a Bite Size<sup>SM</sup>. Now when you select your spoon or your fork you will be able to control how fast you eat. The bigger the Bite Size<sup>SM</sup> the faster you are loading your mouth with food. The more food you have in your mouth, the less chance there is for you to taste every part of what you just ate.

Think about how hard it is sometimes to decide what you feel like eating, yet when the food arrives you do not give your brain the opportunity to enjoy it. This is where Dish Diet Bite Size[SM] comes in. As you are shrinking your dishware you need to shrink your utensils just as slowly and gradually as you did with your dishware.

Let's say you are starting, for example, with a spoon and a fork that are size 28. As your plate goes down in size, your spoon and fork will also go down in size. You are completing your own illusion. If you leave your spoon, your fork and your glass-ware the same size and keep decreasing the size of your dishware, your brain will detect the relative change. This is how we fell for the illusion in the first place. The manufacturers changed all dishware components and we did not notice the change.

Why is changing your utensils so important? It's because utensils control how much food you transfer per every bite. The more food you deliver to your mouth per mouthful, the less you are able to taste it. The less you taste your food, the less you feel satisfied. The less satisfied you feel, the more food you will consume with every meal. The smaller your utensils, the more bites you will get for every meal, and the more satisfied you will feel.

When you finish your meal quickly you are not giving your brain the time and enjoyment it needs to acknowledge that you were fed. Big utensils will transfer your food from your plate to your mouth too quickly. You could probably finish the serving of your cereal in three big bites. Will that make you feel satisfied?

## CHANGE YOUR UTENSILS!

Dish Diet™ utensils are coming soon. Until then you will be able to size your utensils on the DishDiet.com℠ website.

# Food for thought:

**Drinkware:**   Your drinkware needs to shrink for high caloric density foods. This will help reduce the amount of calories you consume. The size of drinkware you use for water can be increased if you want to increase the amount of water in your diet.

**Utensils:**   Bite Size[SM] of your eatingware is just as important as your portion/dish size. It controls how fast or slow you eat and helps you feel fuller without overeating.

**Steps:**   Small steps in reducing all your portions (meals, snacks, and drinks) will help you determine the portion size and Bite Size[SM] that is right for you at every stage of your life.

# Chapter 11

# Change Your Home To Lose Weight

*"Insanity: doing the same thing over and over again and expecting different results."* [18]

Albert Einstein

Everything in our environment encourages us to overeat, especially to overeat unhealthy foods. Sometimes it's the obvious things, like the food commercials on TV, in newspapers and magazines. Other times it's more subtle, like coffee shops on every corner, or larger plates and packages. And the advertisers study our behavior to learn what messages, pictures, colors, packaging, etc., work best to make us spend and consume more.

We are all victims of a massive advertising campaign. Digital photography and computer touch-ups make food look so good, so fresh and delicious that your senses can almost smell and taste it, even from the pages of magazines. Pizza with steam coming off the top and stringy gooey cheese that says "eat me." Beautiful, happy (and thin) people eating chips and drinking beer while having a good time with friends. Even the color of our dishware and our food can be used to get us to eat more. Advertising repeatedly burns these images into your brain: eat this or drink that, and you, too, can be happy and popular. So how are we supposed to resist these temptations?

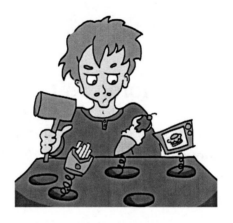

We say fight fire with fire. With so many businesses today competing for your next bite, you need a strategy to combat that advertising. As they blast the greasy burgers and globs of ice cream and chocolate in your face, set up a counter-attack. Fight their marketing and advertising by creating a marketing campaign of your own.

The Dish Diet$^{SM}$ philosophy is to work with your brain to help you succeed in making healthy food choices. By understanding how your brain works, you don't have to be a victim of advertising. Take time to think about it and you'll find many easy actions you can take to improve your health and your life. Here are some tips on how to fight back:

Out of sight, out of mind! Remember this as you redesign your surroundings.

Try not to watch commercials. Battle the bulge with the mute button, or fast-forward through commercials. Watch DVD's instead of movies on TV.

The Food Channel and cooking shows should be off limits for anyone who is even slightly overweight. (You can use parental controls to protect yourself!)

Keep healthy foods within easy reach, and in sight. Put high fat/high calorie foods out of sight. Even better, do not bring them to your home at all.

Go through your house and remove objects and decorations that make you think of eating. Hide them, or give them away. Instead, choose images of nature and outdoor activities, happy family photos, or calming abstracts.

Do not bring snacks into the house. Leave them in the store, especially those you crave. If you do bring snacks home, put them somewhere hard to get. And put them in ugly brown bags or solid containers so you can't see them.

Remove every candy dish and replace it with a book about health or exercise.

Put a jump rope and weights in the TV room. Use them during shows or commercials.

Put a water bottle next to your TV chair.

Chew gum instead of eating a snack.

Cook smaller quantities, using smaller pots, and eliminate leftovers. Food tastes better when it's fresh and you'll remove the temptation to eat more than you need. If you must cook larger quantities to save time later in the week, put the leftovers in the refrigerator immediately, before you sit down to eat. Freeze leftovers. They will taste better than frozen foods you buy.

Do not eat when you are absolutely famished. Have a carrot stick and wait 10-15 minutes.

Do not shop for groceries when you are hungry. Always take a shopping list, and stick to it. Shop right after dinner. Moving around will help your body digest.

Change your utensils. Smaller spoons and forks mean taking more bites!

When shopping, buy more fresh produce first, then the stuff you need for the house. If you fill up your cart with healthy food and necessities, you will not have room for snacks and soda! Does your store take you through the bakery aisle first? Don't fall for their marketing scheme. Stick to your own marketing plan.

Repackage bulk foods into smaller containers. It's best if you can't see the contents through the container. Just label them so you know what's inside.

If your commute takes you past a lot of restaurants and billboards with food ads, change your route. A relaxing drive through the countryside may add a couple of minutes to your commute, but you will get home more relaxed and not as famished. Drive by tennis courts, golf courses, gyms.

Remove labels (if possible) that make bad things look appetizing. You can put your own labels on them like: "Hip Booster," "Waist Expander," "X-Large Guaranteed."

Rearrange your cabinets and refrigerators. It costs you nothing but a little bit of time and you can add more activity into your life. Take a tip from the supermarkets, but use it to your advantage: put things you should be eating at eye level. Things you crave belong on the lowest or highest shelves behind everything else. Make it hard to get to them.

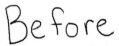

Before

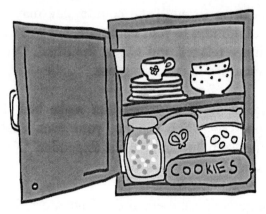

After

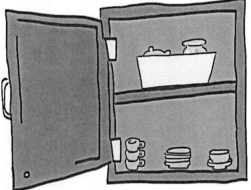

Do not buy or drink soda or juices that contain lots of sugar or corn syrup! You wouldn't put 10 teaspoons of sugar in your coffee or tea, so why would you drink sugar water with some chemicals added for flavor and color? Even 100% fruit juices are high in sugar. If you can't stop, at least combat it with smaller size Dish Diet™ glassware. Another way to help wean yourself off of sweet drinks is add a spoonful of water to a glass of juice. Next week two spoonfuls, the following week three... Small changes work!

If you love to bake, find tasty, low calorie, highly nutritious foods your family will enjoy. Most important, shrink the size of individual portions you serve.

Baking-ware and recipes were upsized. Shrink the size of baking-ware and cut down recipes. Gradually reduce the size of pieces served.

If you order pizza, ask for the small size and ask them to double slice it. Today's small is what used to be medium. What used to be small is now called "individual" in a lot of places.

Does the food call you through the clear containers? Cover them up with healthy images cut from outdoor or exercise magazines.

Beware: Restaurants are coming out with new "bite size" desserts. These are still high in calories, high Caloric Density Mark^SM foods (but at least the portions are small).

Your body has a daily cycle. There are times when you are wide awake, and other times when you feel sleepy. Some people are "morning people" and others are "night owls." There are times when your metabolism is working at high speed, and other times when it slows way down.

Work with your metabolism's daily cycle, not against it. Your metabolism runs at high speed during the day. At night it slows down, so eating big meals late at night will cause you to gain more weight and may result in heartburn and indigestion. If you have to have something at night, make it a small snack. (And a smaller snack next time, and smaller...)

Snacks are controlled with the Dish Diet[SM] as well. We are currently working on Dish Diet[TM] Snackware that so many of our customers request. Until then, you need to gradually decrease the size of your snacks. Always eat your snack from a bowl or plate, never directly from a package. Use the Dish Diet[TM] dishes for snacks – just choose one of the smaller plates or bowls in the set. And, over time, decrease the size of your snack dish, just like you decrease the size of the dish for your main meals!

*"Once you say you're going to settle for second, that's what happens to you in life."* [20]
John F. Kennedy

## YOUR MARKETING PLAN

Take control of your environment. Eliminate things that make you think of eating. Keep only healthy foods in your home. Find ways to include more exercise and physical activity in your life. Eat to refuel your body, not out of boredom or unhappiness.

Your living space needs to support and constantly market to you: "Go for a walk, dance, sing, play, call a friend..." instead of constantly saying "You are hungry, eat this, that looks delicious..." Imagine the way you want to look and feel, and surround yourself with visual reminders (a photo from your youth or a picture of healthy, active people). You CAN do this!

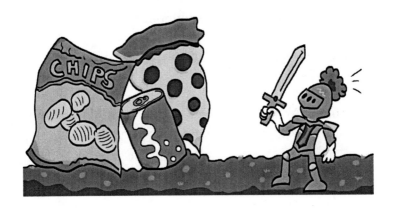

*"The only way to get rid of temptation
is to yield to it."* [21]

Oscar Wilde

Mr. Wilde is right in a lot of ways, but we believe that you can circumvent temptation with another temptation. Substitute good food for bad. Substitute thoughts of active fun for lazy thoughts. Tempt yourself with the right stuff!

# Food for thought:

**Home:**  Change your home to inspire you to a healthy, active life.

**Work:**  Change your work environment to help you succeed throughout the day.

**Temptation:**  Fight temptation with a healthier alternative.

**Marketing:**  You are in charge of your own Marketing Plan that will help you succeed.

# Chapter 12

# Family And Friends Healthy Together

*"All great change in America begins at the dinner table."* [22]

Ronald Reagan

When you have weight control issues, chances are your children will also. Genetics? That may be true for some of us. But for majority, it's the habits and environment we create for ourselves that also affects our families. Are you helping the snack companies to market to your children? The good news is you can help your whole family when you help yourself.

Dish Diet<sup>SM</sup> makes it easy for the whole family to get fit and stay fit. Every family member is an individual with their own weight issues and their own metabolism. A doctor should be consulted for each individual if they are trying to lose weight. Dish Diet<sup>SM</sup> makes it easy for the whole family to eat together guilt-free. Each person has their own optimal dish/portion size to help them lose weight or maintain weight. Here are some examples:

Dad -            Wants to lose 50 pounds, his dish size is 16.

Mom -           Has no problem with weight control, she maintains her weight with dish size 12.

Son -           Seven year old has a weight control problem. Consult with his pediatrician. Show the doctor the copy of this book, or refer him or her to DishDiet.com$^{SM}$.

Daughter -      Teenager wants to lose. Consult with her doctor (see above).

Everyone has their own goals and their own Dish Diet$^{TM}$ Size. They can all enjoy the same meal just by eating from their own personalized DishDiet$^{TM}$ size. Mom does not have to open a box to get her food and feel deprived. Dad does not have to calculate points to see what he's allowed to eat.

In addition to slowly, gradually adjusting the DishDiet$^{TM}$ size of your family's dishware, drinkware, silverware, snackware and portions, you can make other changes to help make this transition easier. Here are some ideas.

**Do not put serving platters on your table.** Serve what you're going to fit on your dish in the kitchen and eat in the dining room. Put leftovers away before you sit down to eat. Now if you feel like having more, you will have to take it out and reheat, which makes it easier for you to say no. Try to optimize what you cook in order to avoid leftovers and temptation. If you like to leave temptation just in case someone is hungry, make it the leftovers of items that have lower caloric density, like steamed vegetables.

Finally, everyone can enjoy their meal together. Dinner will become a fun activity and a place you can talk about your day between every bite. That will help stretch the time, and give your brain time to receive the signals that you're full. The whole family can be together without someone feeling like they are being deprived of anything.

You might say "this is changing how I used to eat," and you are right, but the environment is changing also and we must adapt with it. We all know what happens if you can't adapt to the environment. Have you seen any dinosaurs running around lately?

Each family member will have their own drinkware size and silverware size. You may think that's too much to keep track of. Compare the effort of everyone knowing their dish and utensil size to the effort it would take to measure and weigh everyone's meals. Right now you are all eating from one-size-fits-all: "BIG." Using the right size for each member will help them optimize their own healthy weight.

Obesity among our children is growing at an alarming rate. For the first time in the history of the U.S. children may have a shorter lifespan than their parents. How is this possible given the huge investment we have put into our medical and pharmaceutical system? Everyone is searching for a fountain of youth, yet it's right in front of their eyes and they don't know it: healthy eating and physical activity!

Parents instill habits in their children that will last throughout their lives. These habits can either be good habits or bad ones. Dish Diet™ empowers parents. Finally parents have a tool to help teach their children to eat the right amount of food for them.

The idea for Dish Diet™ started when one of the authors was raising her children. How much should they get? How does it change as they grow? When do you transition to adult size dishware? No one could give an answer. Each child grows at his or her own pace. Dish Diet™ gives parents the tool they've been waiting for. Now parents can adjust the child's portion size as the child grows, in small increments to keep up with their growth.

Another reason why the authors have developed the Dish Diet™ products is to help teenagers maintain their own weight. Obesity leads to problems with self image and many related disorders like anorexia and bulimia. Children have enough problems dealing with the pressures and tribulations of growing up. Weight issues should not add to these problems.

When a college student goes away to college they "taste" their independence. Have you heard of "freshman 15?" That's the number of pounds a freshman in college puts on their freshman year. What changed during that first year away? Their genetic make-up did not change. The availability of healthy food did. Now they make their own decisions of how much food to serve themselves without having the right tools to guide them or control their portion size. Cafeteria style of serving food is contributing to the problem. The availability of so many choices will lead to selecting more different items and consuming more food. The social aspect of seeing other people eat larger portions will lead to overeating as well. They keep odd hours, and tend to keep more snacks around so they do not have to run to the cafeteria all the time. Having high caloric density foods around with easy access creates opportunity for weight gain.

## FRIENDS CAN HELP YOU LOSE OR GAIN WEIGHT

Your friends have a great impact on your life, just like your family does. Your friend can help you lose weight by being your fun activity partner. But your friend can also drag you down if he or she is inactive. When you are analyzing your past, think about which of your friends positively impacts your life and which have a negative effect. Spending more time with those who positively impact your health and well being will help you succeed even more.

One of the toughest times for us to lose or keep weight off are the holidays and the social get-togethers. When our brain is busy thinking about a conversation we are having with our friends it does not have time to communicate with our hands to stop feeding our mouth. We are operating in automatic. We are sipping high caloric density drinks and nibbling appetizers between every line of our conversation.

Eating out with friends is a tough thing to do. Why? We tend to overeat of course! Once we overeat, our "stretched out brain" is asking for more food the next day. So what's the solution? Stay away from your friends? No, your friends are your lifeline, you need them. But if you have friends who will sabotage your efforts in some way, either intentionally or unintentionally, you may rethink how to get together.

If you meet in a restaurant, go to one where you can make healthy choices. Most restaurants will have no problem with you bringing the Dish Diet™ Restaurant Plate, or any small disposable plate. You can transfer the food you plan to eat and ask the restaurant to pack the rest to go. Some restaurants will put the food on your dish in their kitchen and pack the rest for you! Keep some restaurant plates in your car so they are always handy.

Find another place to meet your friends. Go walking together in a park. Your "eating-buddies" can become your best exercise buddies. Play golf together, tennis, even video games are better for your waistline than sitting in a bar, drinking empty calories and eating junk food.

Stay away from buffets if you are trying to lose weight! Buffets have a variety of foods you feel obligated to try. If there are 20 different entrees, you will feel compelled to try them all, and twenty spoonfuls is a lot of food! And then you have to try the different soups and salads and desserts. By the time you are done "tasting", you've eaten for ten people!

Strategies that can help:

Sit so that chips & snacks are out of reach.

Keep a glass of water right next to your hand at all times.

Put a snack or appetizer on the Dish Diet™ Restaurant Plate. Limit yourself to what fits (no refills!) and make it last.

Eat SLOWLY! Enjoy every morsel of food. Try to identify what flavors you are tasting, what the ingredients are, the spices. Feel the texture, chew tiny pieces and enjoy each one. If you are not enjoying it, why are you eating it?

"Slow-pace" your slowest friends. Eat one chip for every 10 chips they eat.

ENJOY YOUR FOOD! Is your spoon used as a "shovel"? Why are you eating so fast? Is someone going to take it away from you?

SLO-O-O-W-W-W DO-O-O-W-W-WN

Can't get a Dish Diet dish? Then use any smaller one; it's still better than using the BIG ones.

Can't get a smaller plate or bowl? Then think camouflage! Fill up your dish with low caloric density foods to cover the "white space". Leave a smaller center for the higher Caloric Density Mark™ foods that would fit on your portion size dish.

We need to relearn how to eat. Chances are, you are part of the generation that has no time to eat. With hundreds of things on "To Do" lists, you must eat and run! Why? It doesn't take that long. Stop! ENJOY EVERY MORSEL. Taste it, relish it. Give your brain an opportunity to smell it, see it, and you will feel fuller faster. Take small bites. USE SMALL UTENSILS or even CHOPSTICKS.

When you eat without paying attention to your food, you are feeding the Fatty-Buddy. When you go out with your friends, eat only when you can consciously enjoy the food. Do not take bites when you are concentrating on a conversation. Your brain needs to know that it's being fed. When you are busy doing something else your brain can't hear you!

*"Do not dwell in the past, do not dream of the future, concentrate the mind on the present moment."* [23]

Buddha

# Food for thought:

*Parents:*     Help set children's habits for a lifetime. Make those good habits.

*Children:*     Can learn to eat the right portion for their size if they know their Dish Diet<sup>SM</sup> size.

*Friends:*     Friends can help you eat healthy and live healthy.

*Eating Out:*     We need to change how we eat in and out of our home.

# Chapter 13

# You Can Do It

*"A journey of a thousand miles
begins with a single step."* [24]

Confucius

Getting the Dish Diet<sup>SM</sup> Program started is your first step on the journey to a healthier life. The Dish Diet<sup>SM</sup> Program is a transformation. Your brain and your thoughts need to change. They need help. You can help reshape your thoughts by changing your environment. As you transform yourself and your surroundings, keep these ideas in mind:

- You are in control.

- You eat to nourish and refuel your body.

- Fatty-Buddy is not your friend.

- "Diet" is not a "four letter word" - it is simply the food you eat that creates energy for life.

To help you believe that small, steady steps can make a difference, think about this:

- Saving pennies and other pocket change can quickly add up to hundreds of dollars.

- A building is made of a lot of individual bricks.

- A mountain is climbed one step at a time.

- A marathon is made up of many steps.

- The tortoise won the race!

To start changing the world around you, go back to your analysis in Chapter 2. What are your vices? When do you have the most difficult time to sticking to your diet? The areas that create the most problems for you are the ones you need to address first.

You know you can because you have done it before. There were days when you ate less and moved more. You just need to remember those days and multiply them in your future.

Every one of us is different. We have our own way of managing how we live. If changing all your dishware at once is too hard for you, start with just one meal or just one dish. You can change your drink glasses or cups and mugs. Start with the easiest changes that will make you succeed. This will help fuel your motivation to make more small changes. Start every sentence going forward with "I can change..." (The sentences that start with "I can't ..." go into the cauldron of regrets to build your elixir for power to change.)

Once you realize that change does not have to be difficult you will be able to implement other small changes and so on. All these small changes will start paying off and be the source of more energy and power for the bigger changes you will take on. When you've automated how you eat you can look at other aspects of your life that also impact how much you eat.

The same steps you have taken to lower your food intake you can apply to other aspects of your life. You can add movement and activity to your life in small increments and as a result develop a more active style. Finding a half hour to exercise may appear overwhelming to your already busy schedule. Taking two minutes out of every hour to move (dance to one song per hour) will be much easier to achieve.

We don't realize that we always look for an easier way to do things. This is our human makeup. This is how the wheel was invented and how the Dish Diet$^{SM}$ was invented. Our natural instinct is to minimize how much effort an activity takes. We will look for ways to optimize our work. For example, have you ever gone to a shopping mall and looked for the parking spot closest to the entrance?

Some people drive around for five minutes, passing the spots that are available until they find one close to the store entry. They did not save any time. They wasted a lot of gasoline looking for a spot that may be 100 feet closer, to avoid walking about 40 steps. Have you seen people drive from their home to the end of their driveway to pick up the mail? How about unloading groceries, have you tried to pack up as much as you can in your arms to reduce the number of times you go up and down the stairs?

I am sure you will be able to think of many instances where you avoided steps, multiple trips, or took a car when you could have walked. You thought that this was your idea. But by now you must realize that it's the Fatty-Buddy whispering in your ear, guiding you there. Now you will need to try to go against the grain of your nature and against the will of Fatty-Buddy. In the old days no one had to exercise! They had plenty of physical activity in their daily lives. Some of us have a difficult time with exercise because we think that is impractical and boring. Let's find new ways of making our daily chores more active. You will need to look for opportunities to add activity without adding time to your schedule.

Here are some ideas:

**Past:**   Park car as close as you can to the entrance.

**Now:**   Look for spot that is 10 feet further than you usually would have parked, then 20 feet, then 30...You may get to the point where you start looking for spots that are the furthest away. (As an extra benefit, you will find that it's always easier to find a spot there.)

**Past:**   Sit and watch TV.

**Now:**   Stand, walk, exercise while watching TV.

**Past:**   _____

**Now:**   _____

How many steps do you walk each day? Maybe you have heard the recent guidelines about walking 10,000 steps per day. How far is 10,000 steps anyway? The average person's stride length is approximately two and a half (two to three) feet long. That means it takes just over 2,000 steps to walk one mile, and 10,000 steps is close to five miles. A reasonable goal for most people is to increase average daily steps each week by 500 per day until you can easily average 10,000 steps per day. [25]

If increasing 500 steps at once seems like a lot, then take a more gradual approach. Add 100 extra steps every week:

Week 1 - 100 steps
Week 2 - 200 steps
Week 3 - 300 steps
Week 4 - 400 steps
Week 5 - 500 steps
Week 52 - 5200 steps

That's 2.5 miles extra per day, and you are probably close to your goal of 10,000 total steps per day. (You may need to go even slower. Consult with your doctor or medical professional for guidance.)

Think about your daily routine. How can you add those minutes of activity without trying? Thinking about exercise and adding activity will also help to keep your mind off food. From now on get a new hunger, a hunger for activity. Get your thoughts focused on how you can add action to your day!

## What if I just exercise more?

Every diet plan that's on the market will say "Do this AND exercise and you will lose weight." The fact is that no matter what diet you try, if you add exercise you will burn more calories and lose weight.

But think about this: which is easier, saying no to a milkshake or walking for 6-7 hours to walk it off? If you really want a milkshake that badly, make a deal with yourself to walk off 1300 calories first and then you can have the milkshake.

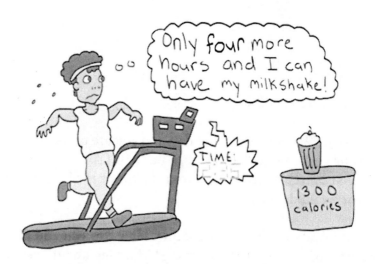

Chances are that your craving for that milkshake will disappear once you know how hard you have to work to burn it off.

One important reason why people often get discouraged with diets and exercise is because they are unaware of the impact of BMR (Basal Metabolic Rate). BMR is the amount of energy (or number of calories) your body needs just to maintain itself while at rest. BMR drops significantly as your weight drops.

Here is an example of a BMR for a 5'6" woman age 40 who leads sedentary life :[26]

| Weight in pounds | BMR in calories per day (rounded) |
| --- | --- |
| 200 | 1650 |
| 190 | 1600 |
| 180 | 1560 |
| 170 | 1520 |
| 160 | 1470 |
| 150 | 1430 |
| 140 | 1390 |
| 130 | 1340 |
| 120 | 1300 |

Why does this matter? Let's look at a Jane who weighs 200 pounds. Jane decides to add an exercise activity that will help her burn 100 calories per day. If Jane doesn't change anything else she will start to lose weight.

| | |
| --- | --- |
| Eat | 1650 |
| Burn - BMR | -1650 |
| Burn with exercise | - 100 |
| Net Total | - 100 calories per day |

Let's just assume that Jane manages to lose 10 pounds this way (3500 calories per pound) in 350 days. She continues to eat 1650 calories, but at 190 pounds her BMR only burns 1600 calories. So lets do the math:

| | |
|---|---|
| Eat | 1650 |
| Burn  - BMR | -1600 |
| Burn with exercise | - 100 |
| Net total | - 50 calories per day |

Uh-oh, even though Jane is working as hard as she did before, her body requires fewer calories (lower BMR). So Jane may find herself at a weight plateau, or even beginning to gain weight. The next 10 pounds will take her almost two years to burn at this rate. Jane, like many others, gets frustrated and drops the exercise.

This is, of course, a simplified example. There are many other factors that affect the total weight loss.  The point we are trying to make is that you need to do both: keep shrinking your portion and keep increasing your activity until you find a healthy balance in your life.

Add exercise and fun activities as your health allows. (Always consult with your doctor to guide you in these choices.) Do it for your yourself and your family. Do it for your mental and physical health. Do it for your heart and other organs. Do it for your 600+ muscles. (A wise dentist once said to us "Only take care of the teeth you want to keep." So, only exercise the muscles that you want to keep working for the rest of your life.)

# Food for thought:

**Move :**     Add more movement and activity to every aspect of your life.

**Change:**     Change how you do things today.

**Move More:**     Only exercise the muscles that you want to keep working for the rest of your life.

# *Part 3:*

# *The Future - Results*

# Chapter 14

# So You've Lost The Weight, Now What?

*"Happiness is not something ready made.*
*It comes from your own actions."* [27]

Dalai Lama

You've lost the weight, great. You deserve to celebrate. Just don't celebrate by going to the "All-You-Can-Eat" buffet. Now it's time to maintain your weight. Dish Diet℠ makes it easy. All you do is change your dish if you start gaining or losing weight.

Your next goal is to eat healthier! Adding more vegetables to your diet will replace some of the higher calorie foods and you might have to actually increase your dish/portion size to maintain your weight!

Some of us can multitask. Some of us have to do one thing at a time. If you like to do one thing at a time, you can shrink your portion first, add exercise next and finally change your diet to get more nutrition to your body. For quickest success, combine all three with the Dish Diet ABC and 123 Plan[SM].

## Change your diet
## to include healthier food choices.

The government's Food Pyramid was replaced with a new image of a plate and is now referred to as "My Plate". The ChooseMyPlate.gov diagram illustrates the five food groups that are the building blocks for a healthy diet using a familiar image—a place setting for a meal. These food groups are: fruits, vegetables, protein, grains and dairy. Compared to the Food Pyramid, there is an increased emphasis on vegetables and fruits, and fats and oils did not make it into the diagram. Hmmm?

Look at what's on your current dish. How does it compare to the recommended proportions on MyPlate? If this is not how your dish looks today, start to make small adjustments and transition to heathier eating habits.

As you are shrinking your dish, you can use these guidelines to help you improve the types of food you eat to ensure that your body gets all the necessary nutrients. The diagram below illustrates how you can reduce your portion size and simultaneously improve the quality of your diet:

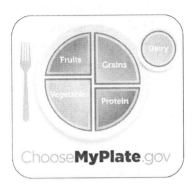

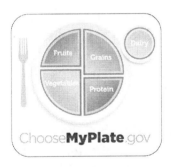

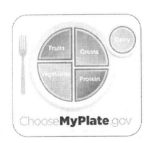

The one important factor that is not addressed by the government guidelines is the caloric density of food. The Dish Diet<sup>SM</sup> has introduced a Caloric Density Mark<sup>SM</sup> (CDM<sup>SM</sup>) to help you make better choices. Here is are examples:

| Food | CDM<sup>SM</sup> |
|------|------|
| Shredded carrots | A |
| Milk 2% fat | A |
| Pink lemonade (A&P) | A |
| Del Monte® refried beans | B |
| Mashed banana | B |
| Del Monte® chili | C |
| Contadina® alfredo sauce | C |
| McFlurry® with M&M'S® Candies | D |
| Camembert® cheese | F |
| Hershey's® milk chocolate chips | G |
| Avocado oil | N |

The earlier in the alphabet, the more of that food you can eat for the same amount of calories. So for example, if you can eat 10 cookies that have the CDM<sup>SM</sup> "A", then you should only eat one cookie with a CDM<sup>SM</sup> "J."

Filling out your dish with foods that have a CDM<sup>SM</sup> in the beginning of alphabet will help you succeed in your quest to win the battle of the bulge. You can go to our website DishDiet.com<sup>SM</sup> to find the CDM<sup>SM</sup> for many foods. Again, this does not have to be a drastic change. Slowly, gradually you can replace the potato or pasta with a piece of broccoli. You can add vegetables into your mashed potatoes that will lower the overall Caloric Density Mark<sup>SM</sup> of your meal. Even though the portion size of your mashed potatoes will look just as big, it will have fewer calories overall.

## I LOVE TO COOK!

We challenge all the cooks out there! Help us transform our recipes! Let's create recipes loaded with flavor and joy for our brain and not with excess calories. Let's transform our recipes to include more ABC foods instead of XYZ foods. Let's downsize our recipes so they look good and help us feel satisfied with a portion that fits our personal dish size. Let's change the entrees so that we can enjoy eating them with the small utensils.

## MORE FLAVOR IN EVERY BITE!

Help us revolutionize how we cook and eat. When we eat a sandwich that is three inches high, every bite we take is a huge bite. A pie used to be nine inches in diameter. Now a 13 inch pie is becoming the norm. Lets say we divide the pie into 16 equal pieces. You like to eat one piece of pie. A piece of the 13 inch pie is equivalent to two pieces of the 9 inch pie. Shrink your baking and cooking ware. Shrink the portions of lasagna. Cut your food in smaller pieces, especially if you are biting directly into foods.

Once you lose weight you may gain interest in a new sport or athletic activity. Without the extra weight, the exercise will be something you want to do because it is fun, not because it's a chore. With your new energy you may now feel like traveling (bring your Dish Diet™ dish with you!), hiking, biking and walking and with all this you will burn more calories than you ever did before. And to keep up with this new metabolism, you may need to increase dish/portion size!

With the money you will save from eating less food, you can get a new wardrobe for your new body, to show the world how great you look now.

But what if you get really busy, or for some other reason, you're limited in the amount of physical activity you can do? Don't worry, just go down to a smaller portion size. No matter how your life changes, you can instantly adapt by changing your dish size! That's the magic of Dish Diet$^{SM}$ - it's the way you can eat for the rest of your life.

# Food for thought:

*Change:*    your recipes, make less food.

*Change:*    the size of your cookware gradually and slowly to smaller ones. Fewer leftovers will result in less temptation.

*Change:*    the types of foods you eat. This may even give you the ability to eat from a bigger size dish without gaining weight.

*Change:*    your sandwiches. Decrease height to reduce your bite size and enjoy food more.

*Change:*    slowly. Gradual steps are easier and more effective long-term.

# Chapter 15

# Living Without Dieting: Eat Less - Move More!

*"Believe you can and you're halfway there."* [28]

Theodore Roosevelt

One meaning of the word "diet" is defined as "the sum of the food consumed by an organism or group." The popular culture, along with companies like Weight Watchers® and Jenny Craig®, focus on a different meaning: "a selection or a limitation on the amount a person eats for reducing weight." The first meaning is neutral – it just describes all of what you eat. The second meaning is filled with negatives; it focuses your thoughts on what you are missing and removes all of the joy from what should be a pleasant experience.

People are getting fatter even as the numbers and kinds of commercial diet products have continued to grow. Something about all of these "diets" just isn't working.

Instead of trying one "diet" after another, you need to change the way you look at your "diet."

Dish Diet[SM] will help remove the emotional negatives of the word "diet" from your thoughts, and replace them with positives: the enjoyment of eating healthy foods you love, in moderation, to nourish your body and soul. Stop letting the FAT suck the fun out of your life and smother your energy. Join other fellow "Dish Dieters" in making a positive change in your life.

Most diets make you count points or calories, ration your portions, or give you pre-measured meals. The constant counting forces you to think about food every moment of your day. This makes you feel even more hungry and deprived. And it does not teach you healthy eating habits.

If you do succeed on one of these other diets, then you are left on your own to figure out how to maintain your weight in the real world. There is a constant fear of regaining the weight.

The Dish Diet[SM] lets you live your life without thinking about food. You just have to remember one number, your current portion size. It makes it easy to lose weight and to maintain your weight long-term. You are free of the fear of regaining weight because you know that you can get it under control easily, just by adjusting the dish size to control your portion size.

# Remember One Number – Your Dish Size

Physical activity is important to good health. We all know that. Dish Diet<sup>SM</sup> does not insist that you must exercise to lose weight, because it is easier to refrain from eating an extra 100 calories than it is to exercise enough to burn it off. We also know that when you begin to lose weight, you will feel like exercising, trying new activities and enjoying a more active lifestyle. While you do not have to exercise to lose weight, your body needs physical activity to help maintain your health and keep every part in good working order.

Other weight loss plans require you to purchase their foods, attend meetings, or join a gym. We believe that the Dish Diet<sup>SM</sup> is the most economical weigh loss and maintenance program on the market. A set of Dish Diet<sup>TM</sup> dishes is an inexpensive one time investment. Of course, with what you learned from reading this book, you can take control of your own dishware, your own cabinets and lose weight all by yourself. But, the DishDiet<sup>SM</sup> program and the Dish Diet<sup>TM</sup> dishware, snackware and utensils will certainly make the job easier.

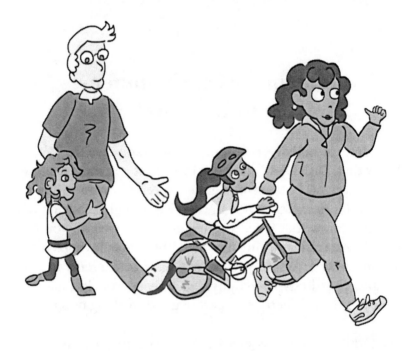

You will find the answers you've been looking for in your own environment. Look at your surroundings and change them to help you succeed. Shrink things back to human size! Look in your cabinets and on your counter tops. Find all the culprits that are making you and your family big and find new uses for them. Your dishware can serve in the future as food platters for the Thanksgiving feast. Your big super-sized glasses may be utilized as a vase for a fresh flower bouquet, but not as a glass for drinking soda or fruit juice.

Replace the dishes in your cabinet with Dish Diet™ plates and bowls so that you always know how much food you need to live a healthy life. So pick up a dish that's right for who you want to be for the rest of your life and just stick to it!

This is just the beginning of your journey, and ours. We look forward to making Dish Diet$^{SM}$ and our products better, to make this path easier for everyone. We welcome your feedback and input with regard to this book, our website and our products. We hope you will give the Dish Diet$^{SM}$ a good try, and we wish you the success you deserve. May your journey be made up of small, easy steps that will lead you to your desired destination.

# Food for thought:

# Eat Less, Move More!

# Appendix 1

# Five Secrets that Most Diet Plans Won't Tell You

### Secret #1

Most diet plans ask you to exercise as part of the program. They will guarantee results as long as you follow the exercise requirements. Well, if you add a rigorous exercise program, even without changing what you eat, you can lose weight. It's a matter of burning more calories than you consume.

### Secret #2

"Exercise is fun and effortless and you do not need to diet, all you need is the right equipment," says the commercial for some new gadget on the market. You see young bodies in fabulous shape using the equipment. "You don't need to change anything, just do this two times per week for 20 minutes and you'll get a body just like that." Chances are that those bodies you see using the equipment used it for the first time while shooting the commercial.

We are bombarded with advertisements and infomercials telling us that if we only had a little more willpower and self-discipline we could get the abs or bikini bodies in no time. If we only worked a little harder. What they do not tell you is that the people in those ads eat a fraction of the food that you are consuming. And if you tried to eat their diet for a week you would feel like someone is starving you. There is always a new diet on the horizon with a jingle claiming that this one will work for you. If you stop eating carbohydrates, or eat more beef, or just eat cabbage, or cookies you will succeed. Everyone is full of suggestions, and recipes that will work for you. Exercising all day long would probably work too because there would not be much time to eat, but who has time for that?

**Secret #3**

"You just need the diet to lose the weight. It's a temporary hardship. After you are done, you can go back to the way things were." Not true! The way you were eating is what got you to where you are today. You have to change how you feed yourself. Until you develop the right judgment of how much food is the right quantity to sustain a healthy lifestyle, use your Dish Diet™ dishware, snackware and utensils.

| Hold the weight | - hold the size |
| To lose weight | - shrink the size |
| To gain weight | - increase the size |

**Secret #4**

Gastric bypass procedures (bariatric surgery) will fix it all up! Snip, snip and you're done. Not true. First, all medical procedures have some risk of complications. And after any of these procedures, you must retrain your body to eat smaller quantities. You need to shrink your thoughts. So why risk surgery? Try to change how you eat first. (There may be other health reasons why you need the surgery. Consult with your doctor.)

## Secret #5

You've heard the claim: these miracle diet pills are the answer to all your problems! Do you really believe that? If it were true, would they only be advertising at 3:00 in the morning? And what happens when you stop using them? Can diet pills retrain your brain to eat smaller, healthier portions? No, but you can do that yourself. Why risk side effects and other health complications? Your doctor can help you make the right decision.

All these diets and gimmicks will make you lighter, around your wallet that is. The flashy ads, great bodies, and cute characters do not tell you the simple truth.

**TO LOSE WEIGHT - EAT LESS THAN YOU BURN**
**TO MAINTAIN WEIGHT - BURN WHAT YOU EAT**
**TO GAIN WEIGHT - EAT MORE THAN YOU BURN**

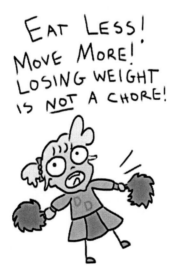

# Appendix 2

# Estimated Calorie Requirements[29]

Estimated amounts of calories needed to maintain energy balance for various gender and age groups at three different levels of physical activity. The estimates are rounded to the nearest 200 calories and were determined using the Institute of Medicine equation.

| Gender | Age | Activity Level | | |
|--------|-----|-----------|----------------------|--------|
|        |     | Sedentary | Moderately Active | Active |
| Female | 2-3 | 1000 | 1000-1400 | 1000-1400 |
|        | 4-8 | 1200 | 1400-1600 | 1400-1800 |
|        | 9-13 | 1600 | 1600-2000 | 1800-2200 |
|        | 14-18 | 1800 | 2000 | 2400 |
|        | 19-30 | 2000 | 2000-2200 | 2400 |
|        | 31-50 | 1800 | 2000 | 2200 |
|        | 51+ | 1600 | 1800 | 2000-2200 |
| Male | 2-3 | 1000 | 1000-1400 | 1000-1400 |
|        | 4-8 | 1400 | 1400-1600 | 1600-2000 |
|        | 9-13 | 1800 | 1800-2200 | 2000-2600 |
|        | 14-18 | 2200 | 2400-2800 | 2800-3200 |
|        | 19-30 | 2400 | 2600-2800 | 3000 |
|        | 31-50 | 2200 | 2400-2600 | 2800-3000 |
|        | 51+ | 2000 | 2200-2400 | 2400-2800 |

These levels are based on Estimated Energy Requirements (EER) from the Institute of Medicine Dietary Reference Intakes macronutrients report, 2002, calculated by gender, age, and activity level for reference-sized individuals. "Reference size," as determined by IOM, is based on median height and weight for ages up to age 18 years of age and median height and weight for that height to give a BMI of 21.5 for adult females and 22.5 for adult males.

Sedentary means a lifestyle that includes only the light physical activity associated with typical day-to-day life.

Moderately active means a lifestyle that includes physical activity equivalent to walking about 1.5 to 3 miles per day at 3 to 4 miles per hour, in addition to the light physical activity associated with typical day-to-day life

Active means a lifestyle that includes physical activity equivalent to walking more than 3 miles per day at 3 to 4 miles per hour, in addition to the light physical activity associated with typical day-to-day life.

The calorie ranges shown are to accommodate needs of different ages within the group. For children and adolescents, more calories are needed at older ages. For adults, fewer calories are needed at older ages.

Source: HHS/USDA Dietary Guidelines for Americans, 2005

# References

1.     http://en.wikipedia.org

2.     http://en.wikipedia.org

3.     http://thinkexist.com

4-8.   http://www.brainyquote.com

9.     Brian Wansink, Ph.D., "Mindless Eating: Why
       We Eat More Than We Think," Bantam, 2007.
       pages 1-2.

10.    http://www.healthstatus.com

11.    http://www.fitness.gov/exerciseweight.htm &
       http://www.juststand.org

12.    http://www.brainyquote.com

13.    Brian Wansink, Ph.D., "Mindless Eating: Why
       We Eat More Than We Think," Bantam, 2007.
       page 30.

14.    http://www.brainyquote.com

15.    http://www.nhlbi.nih.gov/health/public/heart
       /obesity/wecan/downloads/calreqtips.pdf

16.    http://www.brainyquote.com

17.    Brian Wansink, Ph.D., "Mindless Eating: Why We Eat More Than We Think," Bantam, 2007. page 33.

18-24.    http://www.brainyquote.com

25.    http://www.in.gov/gov/firstlady/files/RSW.1.08.pdf

26.    http://www.dhs.wisconsin.gov/health/physicalactivity/ToolCalcs.htm

27-28.    http://www.brainyquote.com

29.    http://www.nhlbi.nih.gov/health/public/heart/obesity/wecan/downloads/calreqtips.pdf

17.    Brian Wansink, Ph.D., "Mindless Eating: Why We Eat More Than We Think," Bantam, 2007. page 33.

18-24.    http://www.brainyquote.com

25.    http://www.in.gov/gov/firstlady/files/RSW.1.08.pdf

26.    http://www.dhs.wisconsin.gov/health/physicalactivity/ToolCalcs.htm

27-28.    http://www.brainyquote.com

29.    http://www.nhlbi.nih.gov/health/public/heart/obesity/wecan/downloads/calreqtips.pdf

CPSIA information can be obtained at www.ICGtesting.com
Printed in the USA
LVOW072148070313

323223LV00024B/676/P